AF823027

World Report on Knowledge for Better Health

Strengthening Health Systems

World Health Organization

Geneva

2004

"Science knows no country, because knowledge belongs to humanity, and is the torch which illuminates the world."

(Louis Pasteur)

"Knowing is not enough, we must apply; willing is not enough, we must act."

(Johann Wolfgang von Goethe)

WHO Library Cataloguing-in-Publication Data

World report on knowledge for better health : strengthening health systems.

1.Health systems plans 2.Health services research - utilization 3.Delivery of health care 4.Knowledge 5.Health policy 6.World health I.World Health Organization

ISBN 92 4 156281 1 (NLM classification: W 84.3)

Design and production: Digital Design Group, Newton, MA USA
Printed in Canada by Webcom, Ltd., Toronto

Front Cover photography credits:
C Cagggero, M Crozet, L Gubb, JL Ray, W Stone, P Virot, World Health Organization (Several photos)
Edy Purnomo/JiwaFoto.com (People around a laptop)
Jareunsri/Still Pictures (Children blowing bubbles)
Peter Bennett, IDRC (Mosquito nets against malaria, African women conducting an interview)
Snap! Mencap's photo competition 2004 (Handicapped couple, Tim and Alison)
Wendy Woo, Auckland, New Zealand (Little girl drinking soda)
Back cover: JL Ray, World health Organization

Contents

TABLES

Figures

BOXES

Message from the Director-General

The toll of preventable illness, early deaths and lifelong disability in developing countries is not only unjust but a critical impediment to economic development and social stability. HIV/AIDS, tuberculosis, malaria, child and maternal health, coupled with chronic diseases, continue to pose major public health challenges to governments, especially in the developing world. In the continuing battle to deal with these challenges and meet the health-related Millennium Development Goals, we have one indisputable ally: science. In the past few decades science has produced drugs, vaccines and diagnostics that have resulted in major advances in the treatment, prevention and diagnosis of many diseases. Yet there is a sense that science has not done enough, especially for public health, and there is a gap between today's scientific advances and their application: between what we know and what is actually being done. In particular, health systems are facing growing challenges and there is an urgent need to generate the necessary knowledge for strengthening and improving them.

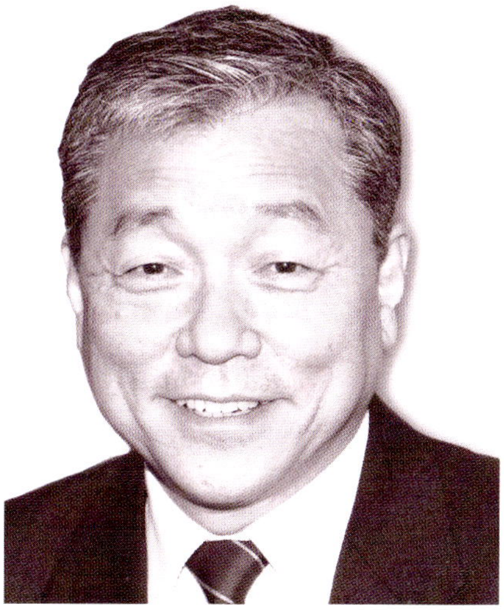

LEE Jong-wook

Through a review of global health research, *Knowledge for Better Health* makes a diagnosis as to what strategies are needed to reduce global disparities in health through the strengthening of health systems. The report builds on previous reviews of global health research by the Commission on Health Research for Development (1990), the Ad Hoc Committee on Health Research Relating to Future Intervention Options (1996) and the International Conference on Health Research for Development (2000), as well as extensive consultations with key stakeholders. It argues that more health equity can only be achieved through better management of health research and increased investments in health systems research. It also advocates using research to strengthen human resources, health financing, information and delivery of health services. It proposes an action plan to meet these objectives that is based on strengthening and expanding existing initiatives, and on identifying options and strategies for future actions.

I hope this report will act as a catalyst for researchers and those who fund and support research, for governments, civil society, international organizations and all other stakeholders to ensure that scientific advances are applied in future to reduce these inequities and improve health for everyone.

LEE Jong-wook
Director-General
World Health Organization
Geneva, November 2004

Acknowledgements

Content and material for the various chapters were developed by a team of writers. Zulfiqar Bhutta contributed to broad health research issues, ethics and equity; Piroska Östlin to gender and equity issues in health and health research; Jimmy Volmink and Metin Gulmezoglu to research synthesis and systematic reviews; Ritu Sadana, Shook-Pui Lee-Martin, Guillermo Paraje, Carol D'Souza, Ghassan Karam, Emmanuel Guindon, Rachel Racelis and the Health Research Systems Analyses project network to health research systems; John Lavis to research utilization; David Evans, Ties Boerma, Phyllida Travis, Mario dal Poz to health systems research priorities. Adnan Hyder, Robert Eiss and Eva Harris reviewed the final draft of the report.

Robert Eiss played a key role in helping to prepare and develop a concept for the report. Advice and guidance was provided throughout the process by Zulfiqar Bhutta, Lincoln Chen, Adnan Hyder, Thomson Prentice, Gita Sen, Jonathon Simon, and Suwit Wibulpolprasert. Tim Evans played a crucial guiding and advisory role in the final shaping of the report, as did Denis Aitken and Ariel Pablos-Mendez. Joanne McManus served as the report's editor and it was produced under the overall direction of Tikki Pang.

Original chapters were reviewed and commented upon by Barbara Aronson, Christopher Bailey, Leonardo de Castro, Tony Dans, Mahmoud Fathalla, Fiona Godlee, Andy Haines, Justus Hofmeyr, Adnan Hyder, Margaret Kruk, Mary Ann Lansang, Pisake Lumbiganon, Hooman Momen, Andy Oxman, Ariel Pablos-Mendez, Ulysses Panisset, Thomson Prentice, Don de Savigny and Cesar Victora. Parts of the report also draw on the work of the Task Force on Health Systems Research Priorities (chaired by Andy Haines), the Task Force on Knowledge Access and Sharing (chaired by Richard Horton) and the Joint Learning Initiative on Human Resources for Health and Development.

Strong and dedicated support for the production of the report was provided by Patrick Unterlerchner, including the development of the report's web site. Iain Simpson helped to edit the final draft of the report. Beth Hochman and Renée Givari made important contributions in performing supplementary research and in the initial development of boxes. Marc Kaufman was responsible for layout, cover design and printing of the report. Pauline McKay provided valuable administrative support. Al Wieboldt, Maryvonne Grisetti, Catherine Roch, Jean-Marc Grégoire assisted in its dissemination. Stéfanie Durivage contributed to the publicity related to the report.

The idea for a report on health research was first proposed by WHO's Advisory Committee on Health Research (ACHR) in 2001 under the Chairmanship of Mahmoud Fathalla. Current and past members of ACHR (Zulfiqar Bhutta, Barry Bloom, Andy Haines, Marian Jacobs, Jerry Keusch, Wen Kilama, Rose Leke, Jean-Paul Moatti, Vicharn Panich, Gita Sen, Hideo Shinozaki, Vladimir Shkolnikov, Fumimaro Takaku, Cesar Victora, Lars Walloe, Judy Whitworth) participated and contributed to its development. Current and past Chairs of regional ACHR's also provided valuable inputs and advice: Mohamed Abdullah (AFRO), Jorge Allende (AMRO/PAHO), Atta-ur-Rahman (EMRO), David Banta (EURO), Nirmal Ganguly (SEARO) and Terry Dwyer (WPRO).

Staff at WHO regional offices in charge of health research provided invaluable assistance by organizing regional consultations in all WHO regions during 2004 to gather ideas and contributions which they wrote up for the report: James Mwanzia (AFRO), Rebecca de los Rios and Alberto Pellegrini (AMRO/PAHO), Mohamed Abdur Rab (EMRO), Yves Charpak (EURO), Adik Wibowo (SEARO) and Reijo Salmela (WPRO).

Many others contributed to the report in many different ways including general ideas and suggestions, identifying and supplying key publications, preparation of boxes, checking contents of boxes, supplying data for figures and tables, and performing research to inform parts of chapters. They are too numerous to mention here and a full list of contributors is posted on the report's web site at: www.who.int/rpc/wr2004.

Executive Summary

Science has led to dramatic improvements in health worldwide. Yet all is not well. Disparities and inequities in health remain major development challenges in the new millennium, and malfunctioning health systems are at the heart of the problem. Half of the world's deaths could be prevented with simple and cost-effective interventions. But not enough is known about how to make these more widely available to the people who need them.

Knowledge for Better Health reviews the current state of global health research and concludes that:

- Much more investment is needed for a new, innovative approach to research on health systems.
- Health research must be managed more effectively if it is to help strengthen health systems and build public confidence in science.
- Stronger emphasis should be placed on translating knowledge into action to improve public health by bridging the gap between what is known and what is actually being done.

The main points made by the report are summarized as follows:

1. Science must help to improve health systems. It should not focus solely on advancing academic knowledge or confine itself to producing drugs, diagnostics, vaccines and medical devices.
2. Biomedical discoveries cannot improve people's health without research to find out how to apply them specifically within different health systems, population groups, and diverse political and social contexts.
3. Health systems must interact closely with health research systems to generate and use relevant knowledge for their own improvement. A culture of mutual learning, problem solving and innovation should be the basis of this relationship.
4. Every country should have a national health research system that focuses its energies on health problems of national interest, especially those which will strengthen health systems. Each health research system should have strong leadership and effective management to enable it to allocate resources efficiently and fairly, sustain human and institutional capacities, generate and use knowledge, and create an environment in which research can flourish.

5. All countries should be able to participate in global health research. Such research should be conducted efficiently, equitably, ethically and with strong public support and participation.

6. Equitable access to both published and unpublished research information is a priority. Such information should be shared with a range of stakeholders in an appropriate format. In particular, an environment should be created where the users of research can access and find relevant knowledge to inform their decisions. The main users of research are policy-makers, health professionals, researchers, the public, civil society, patients, health system managers, and health insurers.

7. An environment conducive to evidence-informed health policy and practice should be created. To achieve this, the producers and users of health research should work more closely together to shape the research agenda and to ensure that research is used to improve health.

8. New research should build on existing knowledge and health decision-makers should use research syntheses to inform policy and practice. Failure to do so may result in serious consequences for consumers of health care and to the inefficient use of limited resources for health-care provision and research.

9. Health systems research suffers from a poor image and has been underfunded compared to biomedical research despite widespread recognition of its importance. Key priorities in this area should be identified. More funds are needed to develop new methodologies and innovations to deal with the changing environment within which health systems currently operate.

10. The culture and practice of health research should reach beyond academic institutions and laboratories to involve health service providers, policy-makers, the public and civil society more. The public and civil society can lobby governments to accept change. In the developing world, any attempt to implement a public health programme without community support may fail.

11. To respond more effectively at the national and global level to today's public health challenges, health research must be reoriented to strengthen health systems through more effective management, by attracting more investments for more innovative research on health systems, and by translating knowledge into action to improve public health.

12. The report recommends that certain aspects of health research systems need to be managed more closely to make even more progress, while building on past achievements of science and health research.

1

Learning to Improve Health

"If you think research is expensive, try disease."
(Mary Lasker)

"What we have today is not the lack of evidence, it's the lack of trust." *(Fareed Zakaria)*

"Between the health care we have and the care we could have lies not just a gap, but a chasm."
(IOM Report, Crossing the Quality Chasm)

Key Messages

- The application of knowledge from health research has underpinned many of the gains in health and economic development in countries all over the world. However, its impact on improving public health in the developing world has been less than expected.
- Global health is currently characterized by persistent inequities, health systems under severe pressure in parts of the developing world, and the growing realization that effective interventions are often not reaching people who need them most.
- Links between health systems and health research systems need to be strengthened to generate and use relevant knowledge.
- Gross inequities in the research process at both global and national levels, along with a fraying of public confidence in science, are manifestations of the global health research endeavour that require immediate attention.

Interesting numbers

1,000/100,000	Maternal mortality to live births ratio in Kenya, where 41% of births were assisted by a skilled attendant. This compares to a ratio of 8/100,000 and 100% skilled attendance in Japan.
6 million	Number of annual childhood deaths in the developing world that can be prevented by applying simple, effective interventions.
500,000	Number of citations added to Medline every year.
6%	Mean frequency of research articles relevant to diseases of poverty in five leading medical journals.
1%	Africa's share of global Internet access; 95% of which is in South Africa.

(Sources for these numbers are given on the report web site: www.who.int/rpc/wr2004)

- Health research should be developed and conducted according to universal ethical standards and principles with the realization that implementation in the developing world has to take into account local context, capacity and conditions.
- New research should build on existing knowledge and health-care decision-makers should use research syntheses to inform policy and practice. Failure to do so may result in serious consequences for consumers of health care and to inefficient use of limited resources for health-care provision and research. More research syntheses should be undertaken on health problems with the highest global burden.
- Both published and unpublished research and information should be accessible and shared with a range of potential decision-makers in an appropriate format. Research generated by developing countries needs to be published and properly indexed.
- Health research should be reoriented to strengthen health systems through better management and more investments in health systems research.

1.1 Why this report?

From penicillin to insulin, antiseptics to anaesthetics and X-rays to magnetic resonance imaging, science has led to dramatic improvements in health worldwide. With the sequencing of the human genome complete, science is on the verge of discovering remarkable new ways to diagnose, treat, prevent, and maybe even predict, human diseases. Yet all is not well. HIV/AIDS, malaria and dengue fever continue to wreak havoc, while new foes like the SARS and avian flu viruses appear and old scourges like tuberculosis remain. Childhood infections and maternal mortality ravage the poorest countries, which also now face an increasing burden of diabetes, obesity and cardiovascular disease.

Inequities in health remain major development challenges in the new millennium and malfunctioning health systems are at the heart of the problem. Countries with few resources struggle with creaking infrastructure, inadequate financing, migrating doctors and nurses, and lack of basic information on health indicators.

At the same time, science itself is facing challenges. Unethical practices in the conduct of research contribute to a loss of trust and confidence in science and scientists, and the overt commercialization and politicization of science in the developed world are examples of other areas of concern. The amount of new knowledge and information generated—mostly in rich countries—is overwhelming but it is sometimes of dubious quality and validity.

Chapter 1 of *Knowledge for Better Health* takes stock of the state of global health research. It defines key concepts against a backdrop of history, outlines current global health problems and challenges, and reaches the following conclusions:

- much more investment is needed for a new, innovative approach to research on health systems;
- health research should be managed more effectively if it is to contribute to strengthening health systems, and to building public confidence and trust in science and scientists;
- stronger emphasis should be placed on translating knowledge into actions to improve health by bridging the gap between what is known and what is actually being done.

The conclusions point the way forward, providing a compass to reorient the health research endeavour to respond more effectively on a national and global level to contemporary public health challenges. The key components of this response are outlined in the remaining chapters of the report: identifying key priorities in health systems research (Chapter 2), strengthening health research systems (Chapter 3), and using research to inform policy, practice and public opinion (Chapter 4). The report ends with recommendations and a plan to implement the response (Chapter 5). These recommendations and plan for action build on the past achievements of health research. They also highlight elements within health research systems that deserve special attention and closer management.

1.2 A historical perspective: two sides of the coin

Discovery and innovation: an impressive history

From the perspective of developing interventions to deal with a wide spectrum of disease and illness, science has been undoubtedly productive: it has had an impressive history of identifying and analysing problems, making diagnoses, articulating prescriptions and mounting effective responses.

Since the time of Hippocrates humanity has struggled to grasp the fundamental principles of science and, perhaps more importantly, their implications for human health. From Leonardo da Vinci's groundbreaking sketches of the human body to James Lind's studies of scurvy, from John Snow's Broad Street pump to Joseph Lister's discovery of antiseptics and from Wilhelm Roentgen's X-rays to Frederic Banting's discovery of insulin, the history of medical science has revolutionized our approach to public health.

The microbial origins of numerous infectious diseases were determined thanks to revolutionary research by Louis Pasteur, Robert Koch, Walter Reed, Paul Ehrlich and others. Building on the foundations of the "germ theory" of disease, public health strategies began to focus on diagnosis and prevention. Scientists turned their attention to developing vaccines, antibiotics, anti-toxins and other drugs that could be used to control major diseases.

Other developments outside the laboratory were also influential. In 1910, for example, Abraham Flexner published a much-needed report that thoroughly challenged the medical school status quo. Calling for reforms in the standards, organization and curriculum of North American medical schools, Flexner appealed instead for a strong emphasis on both biomedical sciences and clinical training.

In the 1930s, Bradford Hill persuaded the medical profession to accept the randomized clinical trial as the "gold standard" for deciding the efficacy of new drugs. Hill influenced Richard Peto, Henry Blackburn, Jerry Stammler and David Sackett, among others, who, by establishing the discipline of clinical epidemiology, made tremendous contributions toward studying disease and clinical interventions at the population level. Their advances ultimately produced quantitative methods of measuring disease which enabled the reliable assessment of treatment outcomes in various populations.

These advances led to a number of public health successes in the 20th century. Three notable examples: the successful eradication of hookworm from the southern United States, the global eradication of smallpox, and the Framingham Heart Study delineating risk factors for cardiovascular diseases.

Meanwhile, Vannevar Bush's highly influential 1945 report *Science—The Endless Frontier (1)* was the prelude to unprecedented investments in basic scientific research in the United States of America following the Second World War. This report laid the foundations for the most important scientific advances of the second half of the 20th century.

Watson and Crick's discovery of the structure of DNA in 1953 heralded a "golden era" of biology. The astonishing achievements of biomedical science in prolonging human life and alleviating disease were further accelerated in 2001 with the sequencing of the entire human genome, and those of numerous human pathogens. With the promise of greater discoveries to come, investments in health research shot up dramatically, as seen in the doubling of the US National Institutes of Health budget and the generous philanthropy of the Bill and Melinda Gates Foundation.

The other side of the coin: more impact needed on public health

Towards the end of the 20th century, however, scientific advances alone proved insufficient to tackle the world's most pressing public health problems, particularly those in the developing world. Is science being increasingly driven by economic forces and ignoring its ethical, moral and social responsibility to give entire populations more equitable access to health care? *(2)*. This concern led to calls to shift some of the focus from the search for new interventions to the research process itself: to manage and align the health research process so that it could respond to global public health problems and issues more effectively.

Accepting the challenge, the 1990 Report of the Commission on Health Research for Development *(3)* promoted a new vision of a global health research system. The Commission made four key recommendations: all countries should undertake essential national health research (ENHR), international partnerships should be set up to tackle priority health problems, more financial resources for research should be mobilized, and an international mechanism to monitor progress and generate support should be developed. The landmark report led to the establishment of the Council for Health Research and Development to focus on ENHR.

In 1996, the World Health Organization's Ad Hoc Committee on Health Research Relating to Future Intervention Options *(4)* outlined a five-step priority-setting approach to decide how health research funds should be allocated. It identified "best buys" for developing products and procedures in several key areas, including childhood infections, malnutrition, microbial threats, noncommunicable diseases and health systems. The Ad Hoc Committee's report led to the setting up of the Global Forum for Health Research in 1998 to address the imbalance in global resources spent on health research.

Public-private partnerships that have been established over the past eight to ten years to accelerate the development of microbicides, diagnostics, drugs against malaria and tuberculosis, and vaccines against malaria, dengue and HIV/AIDS show that the global health research enterprise can be responsive to urgent public health needs.

Overall, however, progress has been slow and much more needs to be done to deal with major health challenges (see Section 1.3). The International Conference on Health Research for Development in Bangkok in 2000 *(5,6)* reviewed achievements in health research and reaffirmed its importance, but also noted great disparities in research capabilities, performance and constraints between different countries. The document prepared for the conference identified four key challenges for health research *(6)*: values of ethics, equity and excellence, sustainable health research systems, favourable research environment, and knowledge production and application. The document also noted that expectations have not been met, that the setting has changed and that the same key constraints identified by the Commission on Health Research for Development in 1990—weak human resources, institutional infrastructure and financing—are still major constraints in low-income countries. The 2000 conference presented a vision and an agenda for action based on equity, evidence, excellence and the view that knowledge is a "global public good". One of its key recommendations was to build a coalition of major organizations involved in health research to promote better global coordination of health research for development. Such a body, however, has yet to be set up.

Four years after the Bangkok conference, it is time to review progress again, recognizing the significant changes in the global health context and the need to continue to drive the global health research endeavour towards addressing the unmet needs and new challenges.

1.3 The problem: current state of global health

By highlighting some current problems in global health, this section asks the following questions:

- What are the achievements and the factors that contribute to success?

- What are the reversals and existing inequities and the reasons behind them?
- What is the role of research in overcoming such reversals and inequities, acknowledging that the primary challenge is getting interventions that are known to work to people who need them?

REMARKABLE ACHIEVEMENTS BUT PERSISTING INEQUITIES

The right to health is set forth in international human rights treaties and the WHO Constitution as the right to the "highest attainable standard of health". This right was reiterated in the Alma-Ata declaration, which was drafted in 1978 at the International Conference on Primary Health Care in the former USSR.

Today, the goals of Alma-Ata seem even more distant than they were a quarter of a century ago. Deep economic inequalities and social injustices continue to deny good health to many and persist as obstacles to continued health gains worldwide *(7,8,9)*. There is also great variation in the pace and level of health achievements both between and within countries around the world. To illustrate these points, Table 1.1 shows regional disparities, Figure 1.1 shows inequities between countries, Figure 1.2 inequities within countries based on socio-economic level and Figure 1.3 inequities by gender.

One possible explanation is that health sector reforms that began in the late 1980s as part of the structural adjustment programmes of the World Bank have not been conclusively shown to improve inequities; in some cases they may have worsened them *(10)*. Attempts to foster equity by targeting services, fee exemptions and free insurance for the poor have shown mixed results. Moreover, the push towards privatization and user fees has sometimes undermined public health systems and public health, and may well have accentuated rather than attenuated health inequities.

Looking forward, there is a risk that inequities will become worse, not

Table 1.1 Regional disparities in selected health indicators

World Regions	*Under-five mortality rate per 1,000 live births (2001)*	*Infant mortality rate per 1,000 live births (2000)*	*Maternal mortality rate per 100,000 live births (2001)*	*Prevalence of tuberculosis per 100,000 population (2001)*
Developed regions	*9*	*8*	*20*	*23*
Developing regions	*90*	*63*	*440*	*144*
Northern Africa	43	39	130	27
Sub-Saharan Africa	172	106	920	197
Latin America and the Caribbean	36	29	190	41
Eastern Asia	36	31	55	184
South-Central Asia	95	70	520	218
South-Eastern Asia	51	39	210	108
Western Asia	62	51	190	40
Oceania	76	66	240	215

Source: United Nations Development Programme, 2003.

Figure 1.1 Under-5 mortality rates by income groups of countries

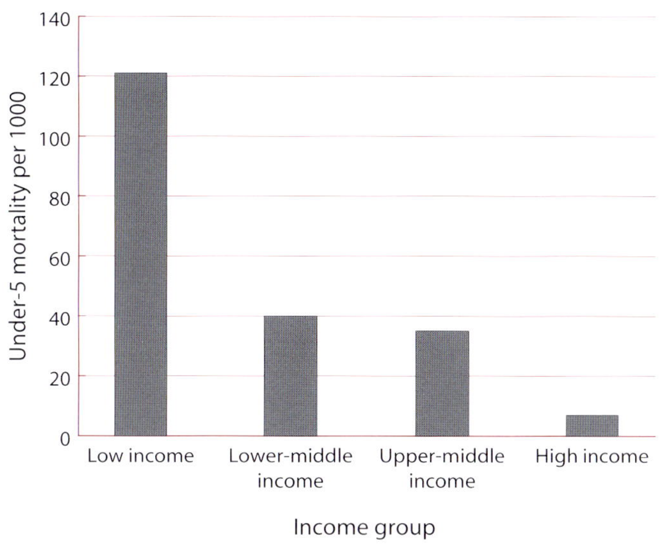

Source: Victora et al. Applying an equity lens to child health and mortality: more of the same is not enough. *Lancet*, 2003, 362:233–241.

Figure 1.2 Under-5 mortality rates by socioeconomic quintile of the household for selected countries

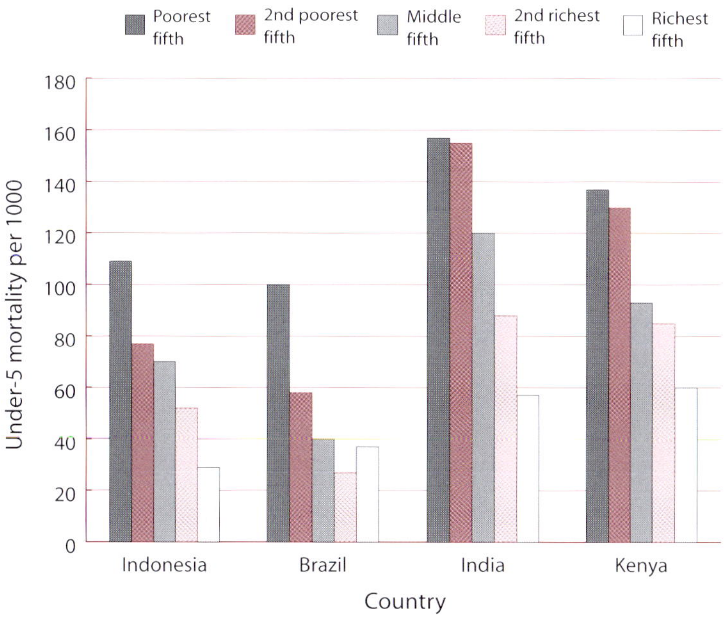

Source: Victora et al. Applying an equity lens to child health and mortality: more of the same is not enough. *Lancet*, 2003, 362:233–241.

Figure 1.3 Maternal mortality per 100,000 live births

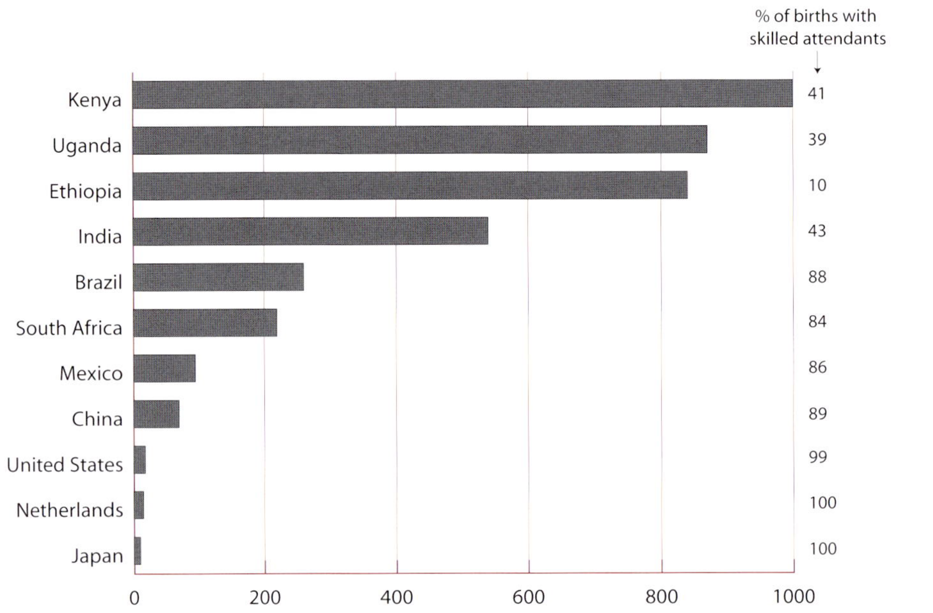

Source: World Health Organization.

better. Rapid progress in biomedical sciences, for example, is threatening to widen the equity gap. A WHO report on genomics and world health *(11)* in 2002, expressed concern about the risk that genetic research will exacerbate global health inequalities by creating a "genomics divide". Will the designer drugs of the future and other benefits that result from market-driven genomics research be unavailable to all but the wealthy few?

INTERVENTIONS NOT REACHING THOSE IN NEED

The burden of disease has been reduced, quality of life improved and life expectancy increased. But as impressive as the achievements of health research have been, they are not reflected in the current state of global health. While one fifth of the world's population enjoys an average life expectancy approaching 80 years of age and a life comparatively free of disability, two thirds of the world's population living in the least well-off countries of Africa, Asia and Latin America suffer overwhelmingly from the world's burden of illness and premature death. Each year an estimated 15 million children—40,000 children per day—die from infection or malnutrition. Average life expectancy has dropped below 40 in some African countries because of HIV/AIDS. The toll of preventable and curable illness, early death and lifelong disability in developing countries from both communicable and noncommunicable diseases is unjust, immoral and a critical impediment to economic development and social stability.

As mentioned in Section 1.2, appropriate and effective interventions—such as diagnostic tests, drugs, vaccines, environmental and socio-behavioural

Figure 1.4 Health research can save lives

(a) Improvement following insulin therapy

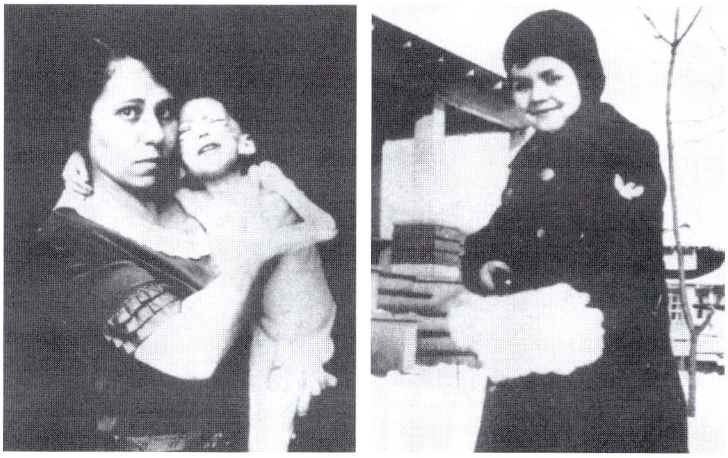

Mother with her child, almost in the terminal stages of diabetes (left) and the same child shovelling snow 32 days after insulin treatment had been started (right).

Source: Wrenshall G A, Hetenyi G, Feasby W R and Marcus A. *The Story of Insulin*. The Bodley Head Ltd., London, 1962.

(b) Improvement following antiretroviral therapy

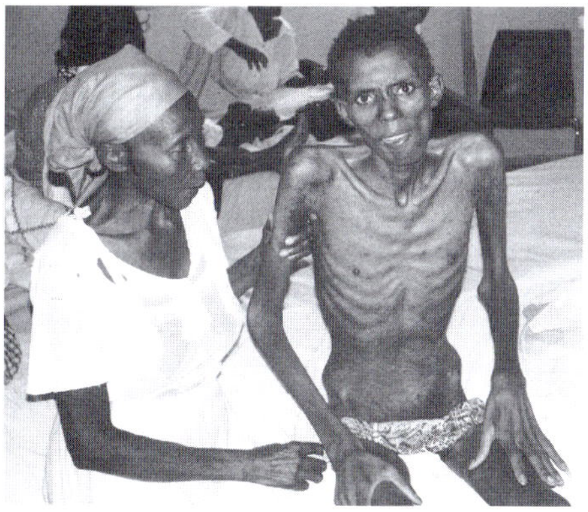

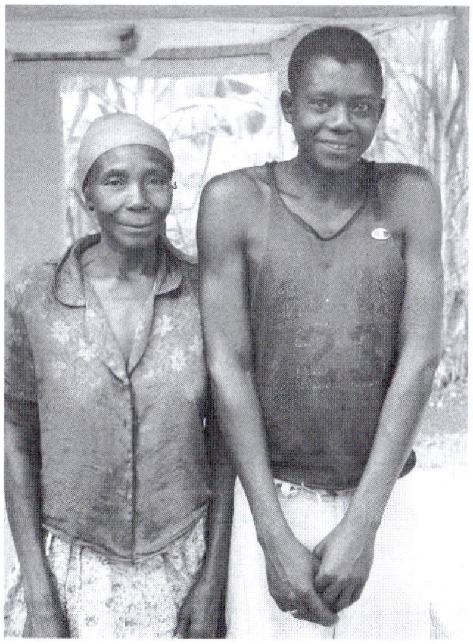

Joseph Jeune and his mother, March 2003 (left) and January 2004 (right).

Photo: David Walton / © 2003 Partners In Health (Boston, USA). All Rights Reserved.

interventions—and prevention strategies have led to enormous opportunities to improve health for all in the last 50 years (see Figure 1.4). Many argue that the knowledge already exists to save lives and improve the health of millions of people around the world. But this is not entirely true: the knowledge that an intervention works is only half the equation of improved health. What is standing in the way of improved health is the knowledge about how to effectively implement and use the interventions *(12)*. This was the conclusion reached by the Bellagio Child Survival Study group *(13)*, which has estimated that almost

Figure 1.5 Actual and preventable under-5 deaths by country profiles for 42 countries with 90% of under-5 deaths, 2000

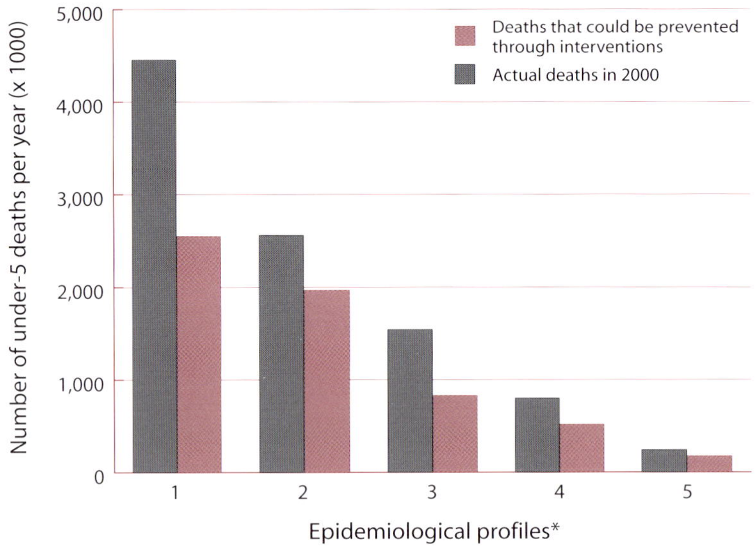

* Epidemiological profiles:
1: Low (less than 10%) AIDS and malaria and low (less than 40%) neonatal
2: Low AIDS and high malaria
3: High neonatal
4: High AIDS and malaria
5: High AIDS and low malaria

Source: Jones G et al. How many child deaths can we prevent this year? *Lancet*, 2003, 362:65–71.

two thirds of under-five child mortality in the developing world could be prevented by applying simple, cost-effective interventions (see Figure 1.5). What is needed to improve coverage is a robust research agenda to explain factors that affect delivery of interventions in differing epidemiological, cultural and health systems contexts. A health system, therefore, is much more than a vehicle to deliver the products of research; it also comprises a wealth of knowledge that needs to be tapped in order to complete the other half of the equation.

Health systems under severe pressure

In an attempt to improve the state of global health, programmes and initiatives have been launched to better diagnose, treat, control or even eradicate diseases and other health problems. Principal among these are the Millennium Development Goals (MDGs) *(14)*, three of which (goals 4, 5 and 6) are directly health-related: reduce child mortality, improve maternal health, and combat HIV/AIDS, malaria and other diseases. However, there are some concerns that health-related MDGs may not be achieved for most of the world's population by 2015 *(15)*. Analysis of the reasons for such unsatisfactory progress suggest the existence of system-wide barriers and formidable challenges in implementation and scaling up because of weak health systems *(16)*.

It is now a global imperative to find effective ways to strengthen health systems in order to improve the lives of people, to meet the MDGs and to prepare for what is to come. Health systems in developing countries are being identified as a key constraint to the implementation of major programmes such as the Global Fund to Fight AIDS, Tuberculosis and Malaria, the Global Alliance for Vaccines and Immunization (GAVI), and the 3 by 5 initiative to accelerate access to antiretroviral therapy to three million people by 2005. The systems constraints relate not only to the realization that inadequate information or human resources may slow progress but also that the focus on priority problems may be distorting the existing systems with unintended negative consequences to "non-" or "low-priority" health problems. In Haiti, for example, it has been observed that babies born to mothers successfully treated with antiretroviral drugs to prevent mother-to-child transmission of HIV/AIDS may then die of congenital syphilis (see Box 1.1).

As the health system struggles to deal with a massive single-disease initiative, and workers are diverted into high-profile programmes, screening and treatment for what is an eminently treatable and easily diagnosed condition, as Box 1.1 illustrates, is neglected with tragic consequences. But if resource-poor health systems are having difficulty dealing with current challenges, how are they to cope with the relentless march towards noncommunicable and chronic diseases?

The huge burden of communicable diseases is well known *(17)* but as

Box 1.1 Health system constraints in Haiti

The tragic breakdown of health systems in the developing world is starkly illustrated by the fact that in some countries babies born to mothers on antiretroviral drugs die three weeks later from congenital syphilis.

This is the case in Haiti, where preliminary findings of a study by WHO, the London School of Hygiene and Tropical Medicine and GHESKIO (Groupe Haïtien d'Étude du Sarcome de Kaposi et des Infections Opportunistes) showed that about 20% of babies, born to mothers in Haiti who receive the Prevention of Mother-to-Child Transmission (PMTCT) package to prevent HIV/AIDS, die. In contrast, mother-to-child HIV transmission in Thailand was reduced to 1% after PMTCT programmes were introduced.

An estimated 720,000 infants are born HIV-positive every year around the world. In sub-Saharan Africa, only 30% of pregnant women are screened for syphilis even though the disease is responsible for more than 30% of perinatal deaths. There are some 492,000 cases of congenital syphilis in Africa every year.

Observations in many affected countries indicate that the epidemiology and transmission of HIV and syphilis are closely linked and that screening for both infections would lead to better health outcomes. Yet in much of the developing world, PMTCT programmes do not routinely include syphilis screening. This is a tragedy as congenital syphilis is preventable if infected mothers are identified and treated by the middle of the second trimester of their pregnancy.

In many countries, health-care systems are severely limited, struggling with poor coordination, the conflicting agendas of different donor agencies and dire shortages of trained health-care workers and medical technicians.

In a country already suffering from such severe constraints in its health system, the ill-conceived integration of vertical programmes, or those focused on single diseases, into the broader health system may hamper what little health care is available already.

This tragedy is compounded by the fact that an inexpensive and rapid diagnostic test and an effective oral treatment for syphilis are available. It is the old story of effective interventions not reaching those in need, particularly in the developing world.

Clearly a more widespread application of rapid diagnosis and oral treatment for syphilis is needed, perhaps as part of the PMTCT or sentinel surveillance programmes for HIV. Such efforts must be informed by more research to determine the feasibility and sustainability of using these interventions in the local context and to address a key health systems research challenge of how to improve the integration of vertical programmes, such as those on HIV/AIDS, within broader health system functions.

Source: Peeling R et al. Surviving HIV and dying of syphilis. *Lancet*, 2004, in press.

populations age and risk exposures shift, noncommunicable diseases are rapidly becoming a leading cause of disability and premature death in developing nations (see Figure 1.6). For example, there were 151 million cases of diabetes worldwide in 2001, a figure that is expected to increase by 46% to 221 million cases in 2010, with the steepest growth in the developing world *(18)*. The prevalence of obesity, cancer, cardiovascular disease and mental health disorders are also on the rise; WHO estimates that by 2020, noncommunicable diseases will account for about two thirds of the global disease burden.

In the absence of an adequate health system, how will people receive the long-term care they require? How can the impact of noncommunicable diseases be reduced if appropriate and culturally relevant programmes aimed at primary prevention, early diagnosis and secondary prevention are not designed and implemented? Efforts to stem the burden will, of course, be important but even with more appropriate primary prevention and early diagnostic tools, will systems be able to deliver these opportunities to those in need?

To rise to the challenge, health systems and health research systems

Figure 1.6 Mortality attributable to 20 leading risk factors, 2001

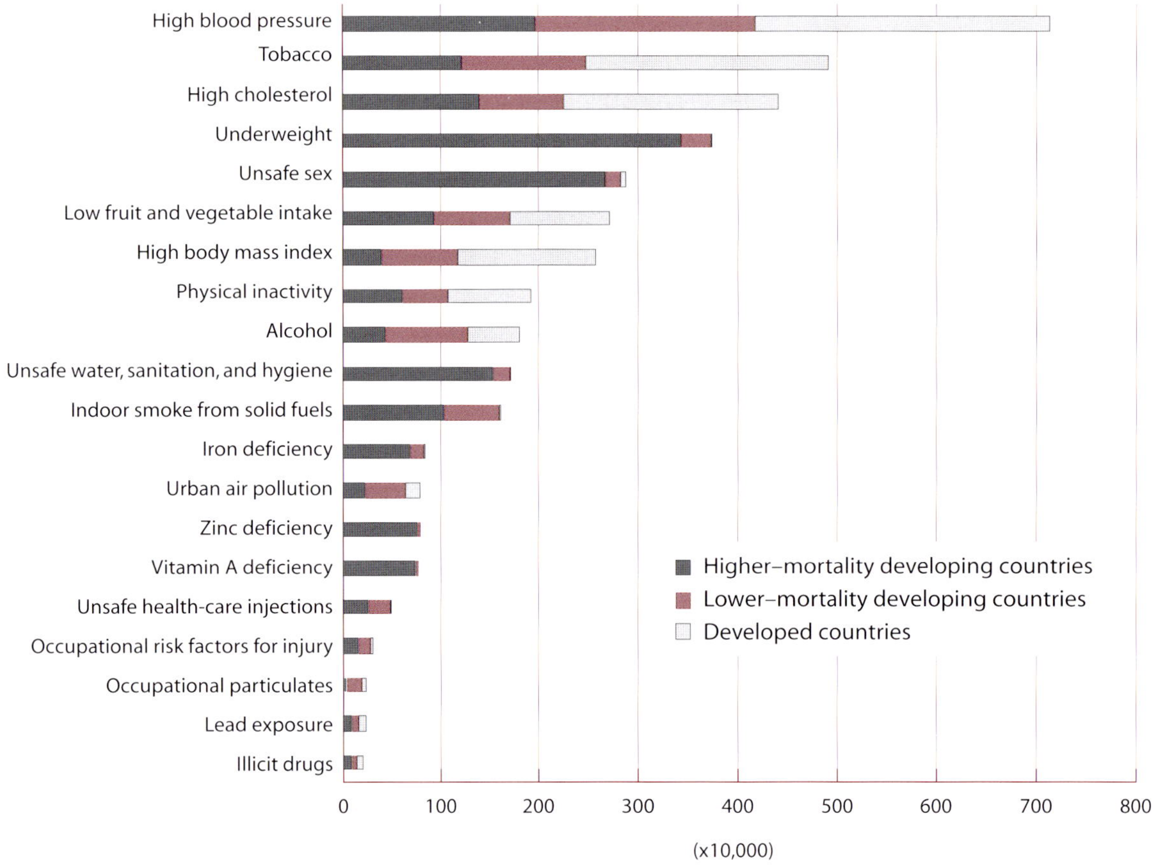

Source: World Health Organization, 2002.

together should move into a learning and problem-solving mode, integrate innovation into their operations and better manage opportunities for future growth and development. There are no quick fixes, no simple solutions and much remains to be learnt. New methodologies are needed to study health systems; new structures and means to translate knowledge into effective interventions should be identified; new tools and delivery strategies that achieve effective and sustained coverage in diverse cultural and economic settings are needed. Basic health information is often lacking or unreliable. It will require new forms of interactions between researchers, funders, policy-makers, health service providers, patients and civil society, and a long-term commitment, political will and support from all WHO Member States. Such interactions have been shown to work at the national and global level in areas such as in responding to epidemics and curbing tobacco use respectively (see Boxes 1.2 and 1.3). If health systems and health research systems were more open to new opportunities and embraced a culture of learning and discovery, progress would be facilitated. These opportunities are discussed in Chapter 2.

This section has highlighted the problem that health indicators and

Box 1.2 Policing disease: Hong Kong's rapid response to SARS

The dramatic appearance of a new disease, Severe Acute Respiratory Syndrome or SARS, in 2003 marked the first global outbreak of the 21st century. Within weeks of its identification, SARS spread rapidly around the globe. Its arrival in Hong Kong, China which borders the province of Guangdong where SARS originated, was hardly surprising, and indeed, the city was soon reeling from the impact of the virus by early March.

The Hong Kong authorities, however, were quick to adopt a set of public health measures to contain the outbreak. One of the key measures was a new joint project called Policing Disease. With little time to devise a new information technology (IT) system to regulate the frightening speed with which SARS was spreading, the Department of Health, the Hospital Authority and the Hong Kong Police Force merged their computer systems into a single public health IT tool. By deploying the same tools the authorities normally used for criminal investigations, the Hong Kong government quickly reapplied forensic analysis techniques to track the transmission of SARS.

To capture data at the point of care in 14 hospitals where suspected SARS patients were being treated, the Hospital Authority first modified software it normally used to keep online clinical records and reapplied this to document all available information on SARS as well as to track the status of suspected and confirmed SARS cases. The Department of Health then developed a SARS Case Contact Information System to trace people who may have had contact with suspected or confirmed SARS cases. This list of possible contacts was then analysed using software developed by the Hong Kong Police Department—software known as Major Incident Investigation and Disaster Support System (MIIDSS) which was originally designed to track criminals. Clusters of potential SARS cases were also spotted and their addresses were verified according to a police database so that their movements could be monitored. The Hong Kong Identity Card numbers of all suspected contacts of confirmed SARS cases were also passed to the immigration authorities to prevent them from leaving the territory.

This IT project was designed to identify and analyse the places where SARS had been transmitted, and to coordinate police, health and environmental responses to this. Its reliance on web-based collation and data transfer reduced the chances of duplicating data entry and transcription errors. Hong Kong's powerful data management system enabled the authorities to respond fast to a rapidly spreading disease.

Hong Kong's transparency in working with WHO and other partners combined with the city's Policing Disease project helped to speed up global efforts to stop the spread of SARS. In June 2003, SARS transmission was broken in Hong Kong after 1755 people had been infected and 299 of those had died.

One of the greatest lessons to be learnt from the SARS outbreak was the importance of being prepared. Since then, Hong Kong's innovative IT merger to track SARS has been integrated into the communicable disease information system for Hong Kong's Centre for Health Protection, which was set up in 2004 to respond to future outbreaks.

Source: www.hwfb.gov.hk/policingdisease/SARS-b.htm

Box 1.3 The first global health treaty is based on research

The WHO Framework Convention on Tobacco Control (FCTC) made history when it was adopted by the World Health Assembly, the governing body of the WHO, in 2003. This was the first legally binding global health treaty ever to be approved by WHO's 192 Member States. Its goal is to protect people across the world from the devastating effects of tobacco consumption and exposure to tobacco smoke. The document is based on volumes of scientific evidence on the risks posed by growing tobacco consumption as well as simple cost-effective public health measures to reduce smoking.

Tobacco is responsible for the death of one in 10 adults worldwide, or about five million deaths every year. If current trends continue, smoking may cause as many as 10 million deaths every year by 2025. Moreover, half of today's smokers—about 650 million people—will probably die of tobacco-related illness.

Much of the compelling evidence for the convention was published in WHO's World Health Report 2002. Four public health measures—taxation, advertising bans, education, and clean indoor air laws—all requiring government action, were identified as interventions that could be applied globally. Taxation of tobacco products proved to be the most cost-effective of the four options everywhere: not only does this have the greatest impact on a society's health, but it is also the least expensive option, as consumption usually falls at a lower rate than the percentage price increase.

Raising tobacco taxes has generally proved to be the first measure taken. Many regions have also introduced bans on tobacco products, followed by education campaigns and legislation to maintain standards of air quality indoors.

The tobacco convention includes a number of control measures that countries are required to adopt. They include: a comprehensive ban on tobacco advertising, required health warning labels to cover a minimum of 30% of tobacco packages, a ban on deceptive and misleading labels on tobacco products (i.e. light, low tar, and mild), and the protection of non-smokers in the workplace, public transport and indoor public spaces.

Other measures the convention's signatories are expected to accept include raising tobacco taxes, requiring manufacturers to disclose to the government the contents of their products and the promotion of legal action to advance tobacco control.

By September, 2004, 167 countries had signed and 30 countries had ratified, accepted, approved, formally confirmed or acceded to the Convention.

Source: www.who.int/tobacco/framework

outcomes are not advancing at a similar pace compared with opportunities for health arising from health research and—in some cases—they are not even moving in the same direction. The following sections look at health systems, health research systems, and at the current state of health research globally as a means of identifying key challenges for future action.

1.4 Health systems and health research systems

Health systems and health research systems should ideally be mutually dependent. On the one hand, a well-functioning health system is critical to the development and delivery of interventions that affect public health and health outcomes. On the other hand, a strong health research system is important for an effective and efficient health system. Both systems are equally complex and chaotic, which makes them challenging to manage and difficult to describe. What follows are working definitions of these two key entities to facilitate attempts to manage and steer them towards the ultimate objective of improving health outcomes.

What is a health system?

A health system includes all actors, organizations, institutions and resources whose primary purpose is to improve health *(19,20,21)*. In most countries a health system has public, private, traditional and informal sectors. Although the defining goal of a health system is to improve health, other intrinsic goals are to be responsive to the population it serves. This responsiveness is determined by the way and the environment in which people are treated, and should ensure that the financial burden of paying for health is fairly distributed. Four key functions determine the way inputs are transformed into outcomes that people value: resource generation, financing, service provision and stewardship. The effectiveness, efficiency and equity of national health systems are critical determinants of population health status.

What is a health research system?

A health research system can be broadly defined as the people, institutions, and activities whose primary purpose is to generate and apply high-quality knowledge that can be used to promote, restore and/or maintain the health status of populations. It should also include mechanisms to encourage the utilization of research *(22)*. The main goals of a health research system are the production of scientifically-validated research and the promotion of the use of research results, ultimately to improve health and health equity. Such knowledge need not come from original research only. It may be the result of adapting existing knowledge to local conditions, of conducting research syntheses or of generating the evidence base for public health interventions. The traditional approach of using research to develop drugs, vaccines, devices and other applications to improve health is well recognized. But the concomitant need to translate and communicate research to inform decisions made by policy-makers, health-care providers and the public is less appreciated. The goals of a health system and a health research system are illustrated in Figures 1.7 and 1.8.

How do the health system and health research system interact?

A health research system exists at the intersection of two larger, complex systems: the health system and the broader research system (see Figure 1.9). This subset of the two systems captures the production of health-related knowledge which, when used appropriately, can contribute to improvement in health status. There are clearly areas of overlap with other systems as well as interactions with international research activities and with the overall socio-political and economic environment, which can greatly affect the transition from research to policy and practice. These various links are strongly dependent on how effectively a health system utilizes health research.

1.5 Taking stock of health research

Erosion of public trust and engagement in science and research

Mutual trust between government officials, health experts, the public and the media is needed in order to advance the cause of global health, science and research. In her hard-hitting book *Betrayal of Trust (23)* Laurie Garrett writes: "Over the last 20 years trust has frayed and our global public health system has been systematically destroyed. The impact has been felt by average citizens,

Figure 1.7 Linkages between functions and goals of health systems

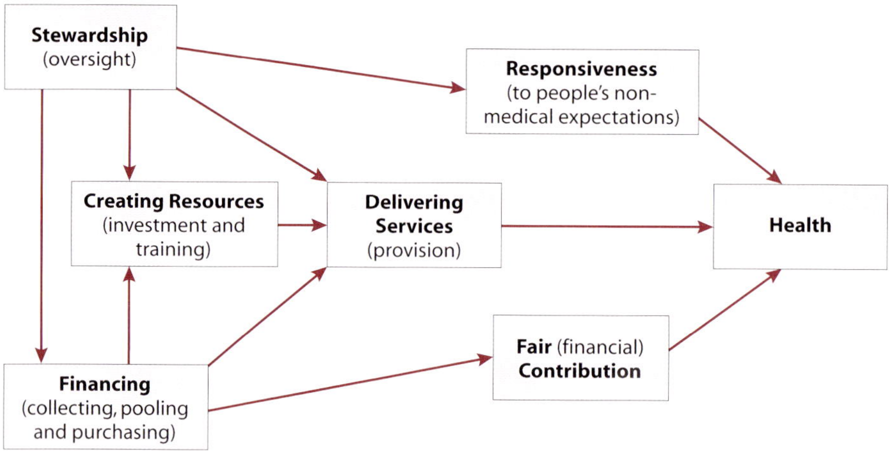

Source: *World Health Report 2000*, World Health Organization.

as a blow to both their personal health and their pocket books". This broken trust has to be restored.

Governments, public institutions and private companies often present simplified explanations and do not reveal the full facts when communicating health issues. Rather than admitting their uncertainty in the decision-making process, they prefer to give the public reassuring advice. There is a growing awareness that this is the wrong approach. Political credibility and public trust are rapidly lost if the public believes it has not been given the full facts, especially on the risks that affect them.

While advances in information and communication technologies create

Figure 1.8 Linkages between functions and goals of health research systems

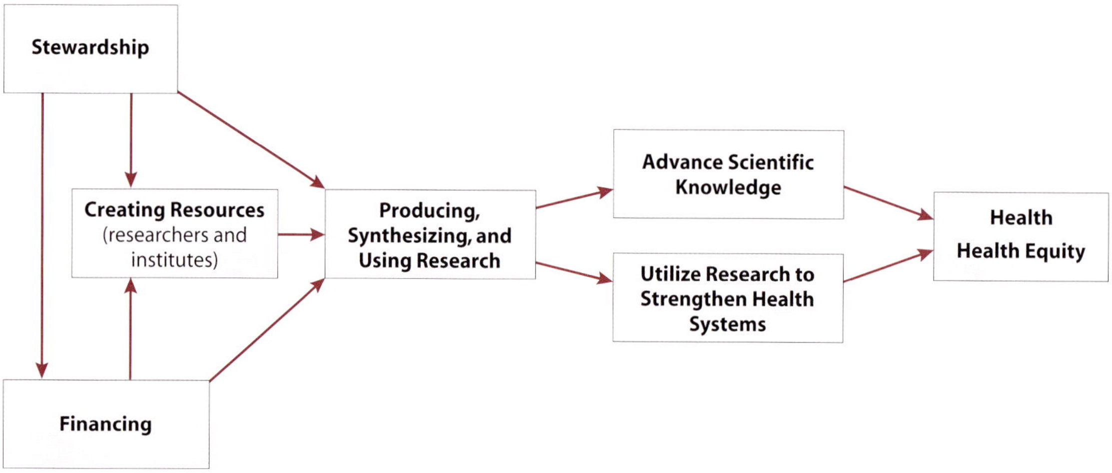

Source: World Health Organization, 2004.

Figure 1.9 Linkages between the health, health research and research systems and the broader macro-environment

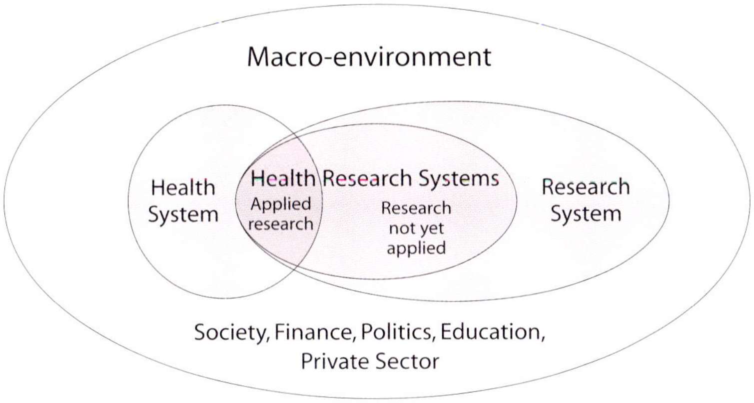

Source: Adapted from Pang T et al. Knowledge for better health—a conceptual framework and foundation for health research systems. *Bulletin of the World Health Organization*, 2003, 81:815–830.

opportunities for people to have more access to information than ever before, the challenge is to ensure that they are enlightened and empowered rather than drowned and disenfranchised by this revolution.

There are many examples of incidents that have eroded public trust and confidence in science and research in recent years. BSE/mad cow disease in the United Kingdom, a tainted blood scandal in Japan, contaminated hepatitis B vaccines in France and withholding information on SARS in China are just a few of such examples. Highly publicized cases of scientific fraud, misconduct and malpractice have only added to the public's suspicion. Scientists' traditional discomfort with journalists and the media has not helped to build public confidence, and neither has the perception that scientific research is often disconnected from immediate public health needs *(2)*.

Nor should we ignore the legacy of distrust. The Tuskegee syphilis experiments in the United States over a 40-year period (1932–1972) are strongly associated with perceptions among African-Americans today that when visiting a health-care institution they are being used as research "guinea pigs" *(24)*.

Increased industry funding of scientific research in universities and other public institutions, academic pressures to "publish or perish" and insufficient accountability have led to questions about whether a research system can be relied on to regulate itself and serve society's needs. The growing interdependence and blurred interface between science, business and industry have raised questions about ethical conflicts between scientific values, profits and personal gain. These tensions have, in turn, raised concerns about the funding of science, peer review, scientific transparency, the ownership of knowledge, and fair sharing of the products of research.

Complicating matters further is the confusion that arises when the experts can not agree on what the results of research mean. Recent reports that have given rise to public comment are on genetically modified foods *(25)*, hormone replacement therapy in women *(26)* and some vaccines *(27)*. Clearly, science does not have all the answers and uncertainty is part of the research process *(28)*. The debates in these situations, however, might benefit from more pro-active management in order to acknowledge the often divergent view points of various constituencies, and to minimize adverse events or health-threatening behaviours.

In hindsight and after a lengthy inquiry on communicating science to the public *(29)*, the UK government had the following advice to give policy-makers: "...a policy of openness is the correct approach. When responding to public or media demand for advice, the government should resist the temptation of attempting to appear to have all the answers in a situation of uncertainty. We believe that food scares and vaccine scares thrive on the belief that the Government is withholding information. If doubts are openly expressed and publicly explored, the public are capable of responding rationally and are more likely to accept reassurance and advice if and when it comes".

A health research system should build public trust in itself and its products by effectively communicating benefits as well as risks and uncertainties (see Box 1.4). Unfortunately, this ability to communicate with the public is one of the weakest attributes of most governments and health researchers. This needs to change. It is vital to obtain society's support for the research process. This is an essential, explicit and important objective of public health research. After all, it is the public (as taxpayers and philanthropists) who foot a large part of the bill for research. Health research is a multidisciplinary activity which exists at national, regional and global levels and it requires large-scale public investment. And with the public's support much can be accomplished. For example, the concerted efforts of public representatives and civic leaders led to the setting up of the US National Institutes of Health, which is now the biggest funder of health research in the world. This synergy between civil society and health research is one important factor that can influence both the demand and supply of essential health research in developing countries.

Given the importance of linking health research and its application to public health, representatives of civil society should participate in setting the research agenda, in major health policy decisions and in the design, implementation and evaluation of pubic health programmes. The March of Dimes Foundation's active support in the large-scale Salk polio vaccine trials is an example of civil society and researchers working together *(30)*. More recently, the field of HIV/AIDS research has demonstrated the

Box 1.4 Important lessons for governments on developing better risk communications

- To establish credibility it is necessary to generate trust.
- Trust can only be generated by openness.
- Openness requires recognition of uncertainty, where it exists.
- The public should be trusted to respond rationally to openness.
- The importance of precautionary measures should not be played down on the grounds that the risk is unproven.
- Scientific investigation of risk should be open and transparent.
- The advice and reasoning of advisory committees should be made public.
- The trust that the public has in scientists, experts and professionals, such as chief medical officers, is precious and should not be put at risk.
- Any advice to the public from such experts and advisory committees should be, and should be seen to be, objective and independent of government and political influence.

Source: World Health Report 2002, World Health Organization.

positive impact of engaging the public in the research process. In the United States and elsewhere, cooperation between researchers and at-risk or affected populations led to innovative research protocols and considerable public support for research.

But such cooperation between funders, the research community and civil society has neither been easy nor timely and it is still the exception rather than the rule. For example, public concern and consternation over HIV treatment trials in developing countries contributed to the development of initiatives to inject resources into global AIDS programmes, and to a global debate about drug patents, drug prices and access to medicine. This, in turn, led to important first steps to making antiretrovirals available to millions of people who could not afford them before.

So whether it is adversarial or in the spirit of cooperation, public involvement can reap positive, beneficial changes that research alone can not accomplish. As the case of AIDS and antiretrovirals suggest, relevant knowledge generated from research is necessary but not sufficient to tackle difficult and complex problems. Involvement of civil society and political commitment are also necessary. "The triangle that moves the mountain" is a concept developed by Thailand's Professor Prawase Wasi *(31)* to represent the idea that addressing complex problems requires not only researchers. They must work together with policy-makers, politicians, the media, consumers and civil society towards a common goal and equally share power, influence and responsibility (see Figure 1.10).

Inequities in the research process

Financing health research

An estimated 10% of the more than US$70 billion spent annually on health research (within and between countries) by the public and private sectors is used for research into 90% of the world's health problems *(32)*. This is known as the "10/90 gap". Such a gap and other inequities in health research may lead to inaccuracies in assessing the disease burden of populations or population groups, thus contributing to continued disparities in health. The Commission

Figure 1.10 Triangle that moves the mountain

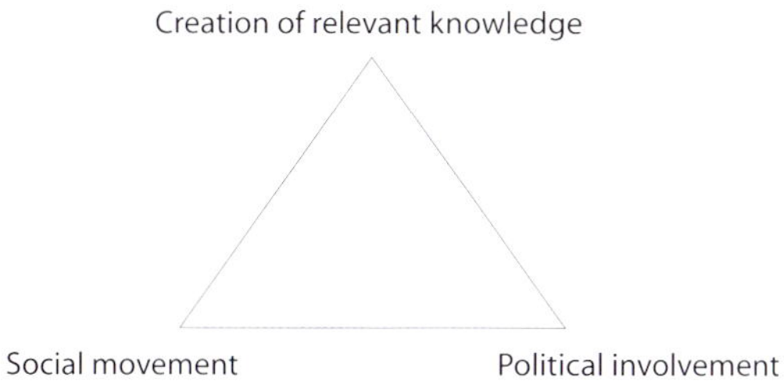

Source: Wasi P. *Triangle that moves the mountain*. Bangkok, Thailand, Health Systems Research Institute, 2000.

on Macroeconomics and Health *(33)* underscored one of the key problems by concluding in 2001 that there were no economic incentives for private sector investment to research diseases that affect the least-developed countries. Though it recommended increased investments to redress this gap and promoted more research on neglected diseases, the health inequality between developed and developing countries remains the single greatest public health problem.

Persistent inequities in setting the research agenda

Given that most developing countries do not have an adequate number of researchers or adequately equipped research institutes, they can not ensure that the research that has been conducted meets their needs. Health research in developing countries is often the result of collaborative partnerships where the foreign donor agency or funder usually has more power in deciding the research agenda. This can skew research into areas that are not priority health problems for the local population. Moreover, biomedical and clinical research in both developed and developing countries are increasingly being funded and controlled by pharmaceutical and biotechnology companies. This may result in a situation where the drug maker's product portfolio rarely addresses the health priorities of the developing country where the research is being carried out. Another concern is that such collaborations divert already extremely limited qualified staff away from research on more nationally relevant problems.

Some progress, however, has been made. As mentioned previously (see Section 1.2), WHO's Ad Hoc Committee on Health Research Relating to Future Intervention Options *(4)* outlined a five-step priority setting approach to decide how health research funds should be allocated in key areas of concern to developing countries. The Council for Health Research and Development and the Global Forum for Health Research subsequently refined and applied such priority setting tools *(34,35)*. The Global Forum has also implemented a number of initiatives based on these priorities, including those on health systems research, public-private partnerships, cardiovascular disease in developing countries, road traffic injuries and child health research.

Another important dimension of inequity in setting the research agenda is the overwhelming dominance of biomedical and clinical research compared to research into the social determinants of health and health systems research. One estimate was that less than 0.1% of total health expenditure is spent on health systems research in low-income countries (32). This issue will be revisited in Chapter 2.

Gender bias in health research

Clinical research has generally excluded female subjects from study populations because it is believed the menstrual cycle introduces a potentially confounding variable. Women are also excluded because of fears that experimental treatments or drugs may affect female fertility and expose fetuses to unknown risks. The consequences of interpreting research results based on studies only involving men as universally valid, without convincing evidence that they apply to women, may be harmful to women.

Although the proportion of women among medical students and faculty members at all levels in the world has increased steadily in recent years, their representation in decision-making bodies such as research funding committees and research advisory boards has not increased accordingly (see Figure 1.11). Women also tend to be under-represented on the editorial boards of scientific journals *(36)*. There is also differential treatment of female scientists in terms of career opportunities, salary, and obtaining research funds and post-doctoral fellowships. In the developing world, organizations like the Third World Organization for Women in Science (TWOWS), which is part of the Third World Academy of Science, are committed to strengthening the role of women in the development process and promoting their representation in scientific and technological leadership roles.

Inequities in knowledge publication

Given the 10/90 resource gap in health research—an issue brought to the fore by the Global Forum for Health Research *(32)*—it is not surprising that more than 90% of scientific publications in health research are published by researchers in the developed world. There is widespread systematic bias in medical journals against diseases that dominate the least-developed regions of the world. A recent editorial in the *Lancet (37)* stated that research papers on developing world problems were much less likely to get published. A survey of five leading general medical journals in 2001 found that the frequency of research articles relevant to diseases of poverty was low—zero for *Annals of*

Figure 1.11 Membership of WHO expert advisory panels by gender, 1996–2002

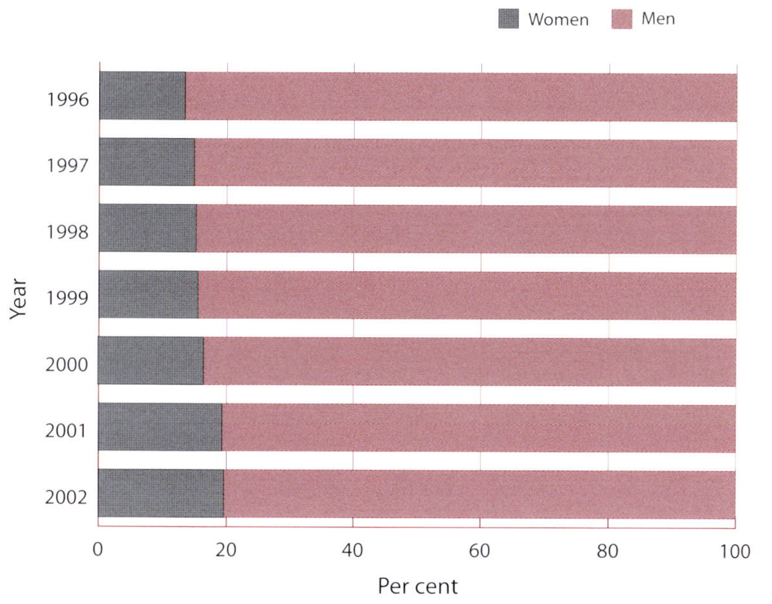

Source: Östlin P, Sen G, George A. Paying attention to gender and poverty in health research: content and process issues. *Bulletin of the World Health Organization*, 82;740–745.

Internal Medicine, 2% for *Journal of the American Medical Association*, 4% for the *New England Journal of Medicine*, 6% for the *British Medical Journal*, and 16% for the *Lancet*. Also, few papers are published that involve research on noncommunicable diseases in developing countries (see Figure 1.12).

Although the values that influence decisions about the selection of content for medical journals are largely determined by priorities in science, public health and commerce, the composition of editorial boards is important too, as it sends a signal to authors and readers about a journal's interests. An improvement in the representation of scientists from developing countries on the editorial boards of major medical journals may improve the attention given to health challenges in these countries.

Divide in access to information

The peer reviewed scientific and health-care literature exists in the form of journals. Access to local, regional and international journals is especially important for researchers and systematic reviewers. Researchers in rich countries enjoy relatively easy access to research information but for many researchers in resource-poor environments, access to available research is far from easy. Internet access remains poor (see below) and few researchers or institutions in developing countries can afford the high cost of journal subscriptions (print

Figure 1.12 Number of authors from regions and countries publishing or co-publishing papers on chronic diseases or their major risk factors, 1990–1993 and 2000–2003

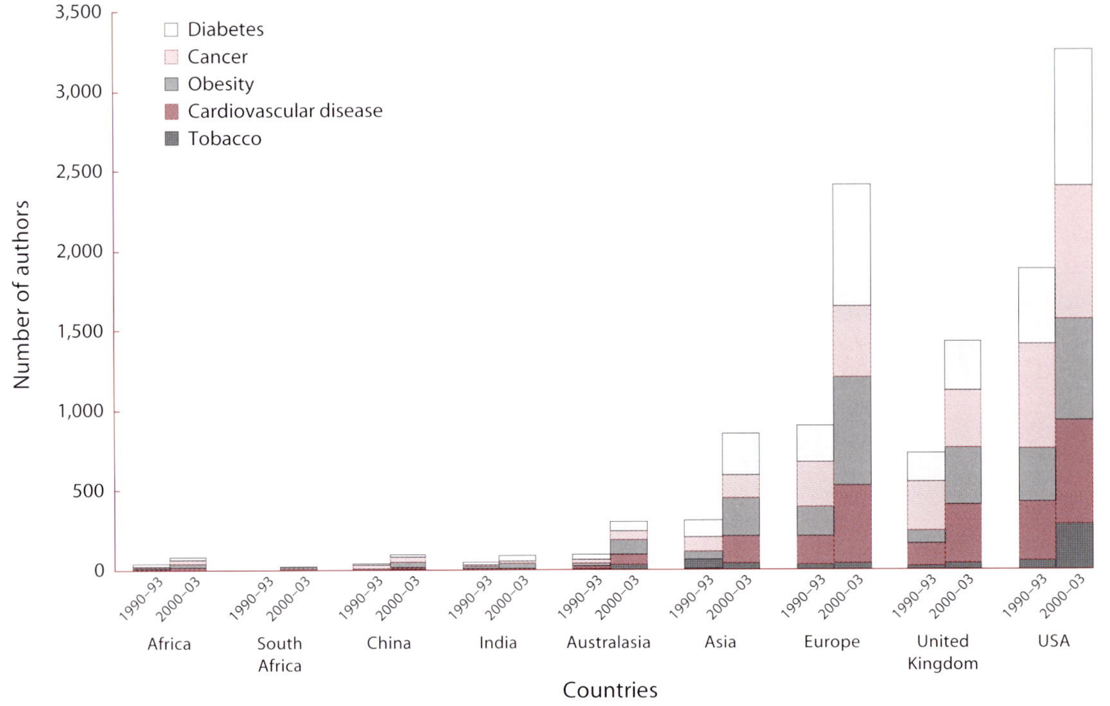

Source: D Yach, S Glover, N Cohen. Personal communication.

or electronic). The divide in access is exacerbated by the massive increase in the number of scientific articles on health published each year (see Figure 1.13)

In September 2000, in its statement on the right of access to information and communication, the Millennium Assembly of the United Nations emphasized the importance of information in relation to learning, research and debates. While the electronic revolution is providing scientists and health

Figure 1.13 Articles indexed in PubMed, 1950–1999

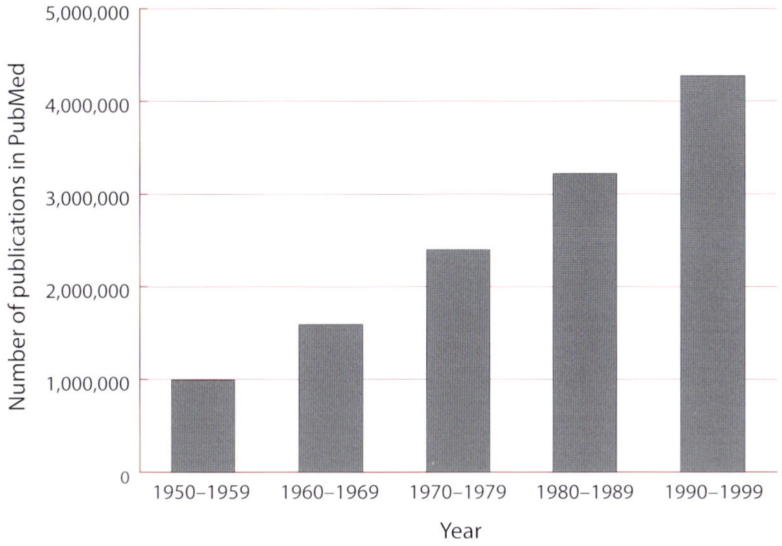

Source: Data supplied by P Sieving, M Ryan, B Otterson. National Institutes of Health Library, Bethesda, MD, USA.

Figure 1.14 Global Internet access, 2002

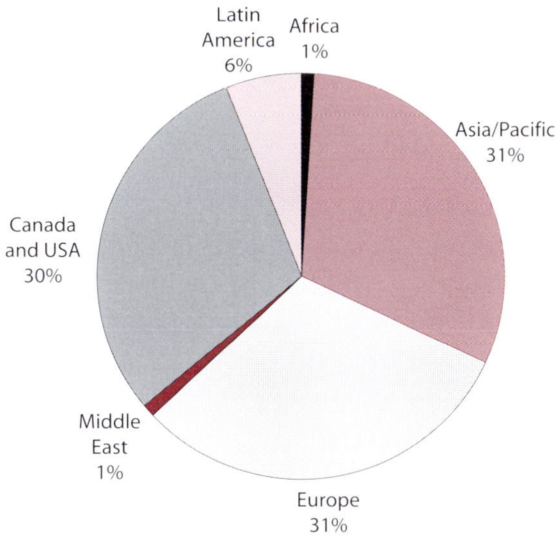

Source: Nua Internet surveys.

workers in the developed world with unprecedented access to information, the same groups in the developing world may have very limited access to any information apart from outdated textbooks *(38)*. Because many scientific journals now are purely electronic, many researchers in poor countries do not have access to them. Africa only has 1% of global Internet access and, of this, 95% is in South Africa (see Figure 1.14).

Research favours generating new knowledge over assimilating what is already known

Research to date has focused on the generation of new knowledge but has tended to neglect the role and contribution of existing knowledge. This neglect has led to inefficient use of limited resources for research and missed opportunities for achieving health gains. Knowledge depends as much on the evaluation of existing research as it does on the generation of new research. This is because the results of an individual study, however interesting, cannot be relied upon when making informed decisions about health care. What should be determined is how the results of a particular study compare with other studies relating to the same question.

Science is meant to be cumulative. New research should ideally be interpreted within the context of an existing body of scientific knowledge. Research synthesis, which is the application of this principle in practice, is not a new concept. At a meeting of the British Association for the Advancement of Science in 1884, Lord Rayleigh, a Professor of Physics at Cambridge University, stated: "Two processes are thus at work side by side, the reception of new material and the digestion and assimilation of the old; and as both are essential we may spare ourselves the discussion of their relative importance." His remarks are just as relevant today.

Systematic reviews have become the "gold standard" for assimilating and digesting research *(39,40)*. By applying a rigorous and transparent methodology to research synthesis, systematic reviews reduce systematic error (bias) and random error (the play of chance) that bedevil the review process. They are increasingly being used to inform health-care decisions such as whether a particular health-care intervention should be used or not. The flowchart in Figure 1.15 illustrates how a systematic review can contribute to saving lives, respecting resources and spurring research.

But despite their central role in a knowledge-based health system, and despite the skill and time they require, systematic reviews do not attract anywhere near the same level of academic recognition or public attention as primary (especially biomedical) research. They are largely performed by researchers and health-care professionals who volunteer their time outside their main work activities, few of whom are based in developing countries. As a result, the number of published systematic reviews is still relatively small, the coverage of different diseases and other aspects of health care is uneven, and few reviews are related to diseases with a high global burden *(41)* (see Figure 1.16).

Figure 1.15 Value and impact of systematic reviews

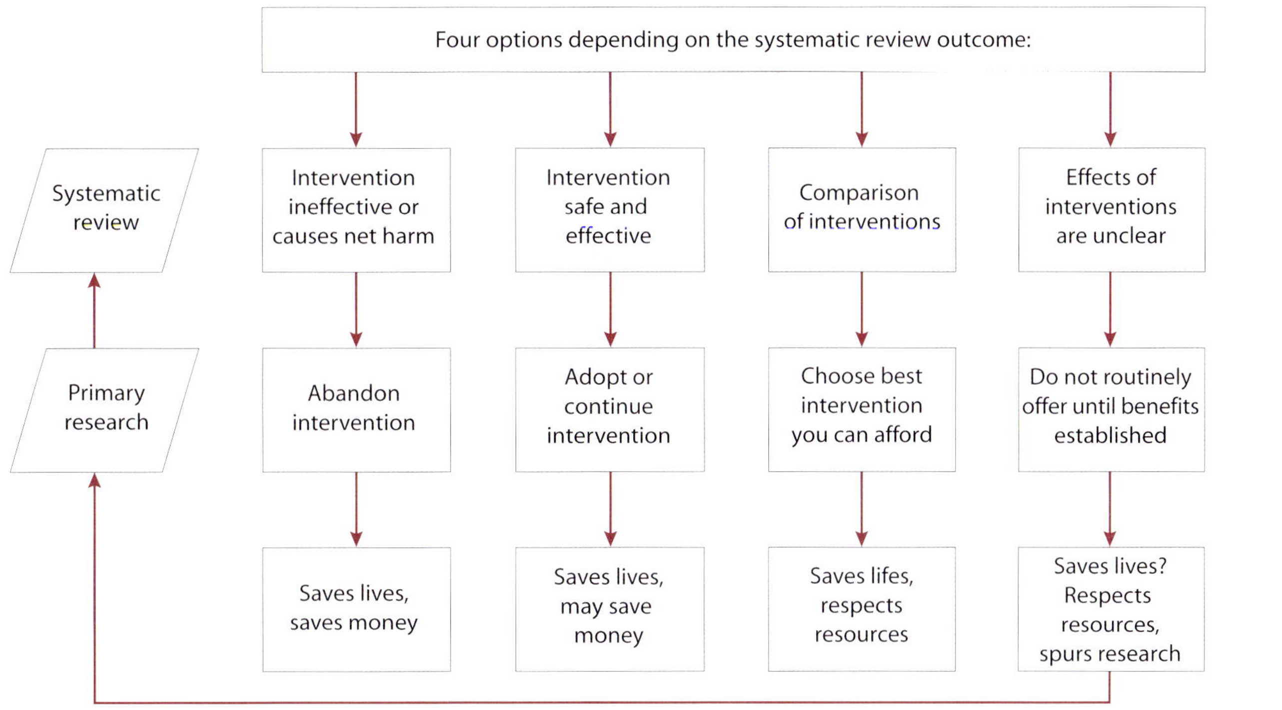

Source: Volmink J, Murphy C, Woldehanna S. Towards an evidence-based approach to decision making. In: *Making childbirth safer through evidence-based care*. Global Health Council, Washington DC, USA, 2002.

Figure 1.16 Number and proportion of systematic reviews in developed and developing countries

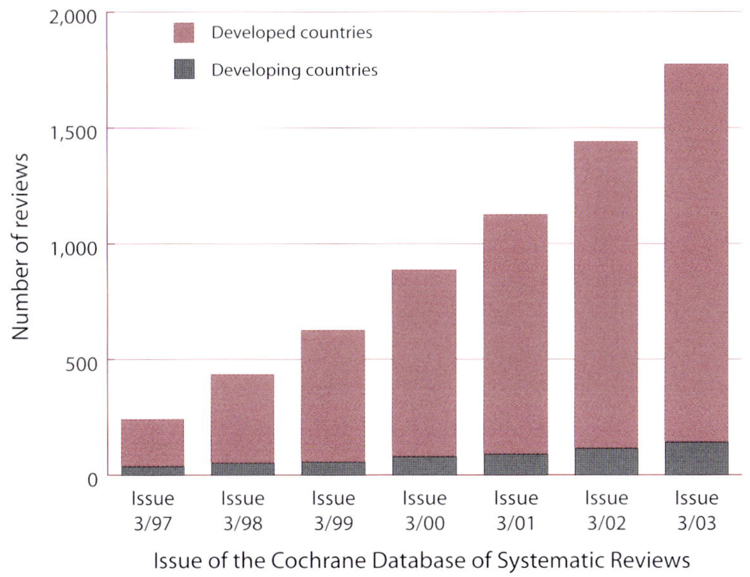

Source: Volmink J. Personal communication (based on analysis by P Alderson, UK Cochrane Centre on behalf of South African Cochrane Centre).

Lack of openness and accountability impairs ability to draw conclusions from research

The diversity of funding sources for research, and the settings in which research takes place, calls for across-the-board policies that provide appropriate guidelines on making research results known. A clinical trial result may not be published because a company abandons its plans to bring the drug to market. Publication may not be pursued because the results are negative or neutral, or because the trial was stopped before completion. Whatever the reason, if study results are never made public, no knowledge is gained. The serious problem of "publication bias" was identified more than 10 years ago *(42)*. Recent concerns about this bias, however, have been brought to the public's attention and a clear approach to dealing with the problem is necessary.

The problem came to the forefront once again in June 2004 regarding lack of information on clinical trial results for an antidepressant *(43,44)*. Following the highlighting of these concerns by the media *(45,46)*, a strong call was made for improved transparency and access to the results of clinical trials *(47,48)*.

Information about a drug that does not demonstrate efficacy in a controlled trial or one that demonstrates significant hazards is important for those making health-care decisions. If scientific findings are not reported or published, there may be implications for compromising the health and safety of patients, and causing inefficient use of resources.

To ensure that systematic reviews and other kinds of research syntheses are unbiased, or at least that the potential for bias can be estimated, the possibility of all controlled trials being accessible on an international trial register needs serious consideration *(49,50)*. Not having access to all valid research can seriously jeopardize the quality and reliability of a systematic review. It can delay implementation of effective interventions or prolong the use of ineffective or even harmful interventions. But accessing such information is often difficult. With increasing interest in commercialization of research findings, sometimes coupled with limited government funding for research, scientists are often the recipients of research grants from the commercial sector. In some cases, they may not have complete control on how the research results are used.

Moreover, the confidence and trust of the public and the health profession may be affected if there should be indications that evidence of harm or overstatement of benefits were not fully disclosed due to commercial pressures. Ethical health research principles demand timely and accurate reporting of research results to study participants, researchers and all potential users of research. It follows that human research undertaken with the full knowledge that the study results may not be in the public domain can be considered unethical.

Unresolved issues surrounding the ethics of research in developing countries

While the fundamental principles of ethical health research, such as community participation, informed consent, and shared benefits and burdens, remain sacrosanct, other issues, such as standards of care and prior agreements, merit greater debate *(51,52)*. International guidelines such as the Declaration of Helsinki and the guidelines issued by the Council for International Organizations of Medical Sciences *(53)* have significant influence on international funding agencies and the pharmaceutical industry and form a cornerstone of research ethics in much of the developing world. The problem is that the stringent application of certain criteria in these guidelines would effectively stop much-needed public health and epidemiological research. Consider, for example, the issue of standards of care. Exactly what constitutes the standard of care is open to interpretation: it can be interpreted as the global standard of care, or the locally existing standard, or a general standard of care in the research setting, including aspects of sustainability.

A trial in Gadchiroli, India, is an interesting case in point. Researchers undertook an evaluation of home neonatal care with community-based health workers administering an oral antibiotic called trimethoprim-sulfamethoxazole and twice-daily gentamicin to newborn infants with suspected sepsis. After an elaborate scientific and ethical review process, the community agreed to participate in the study despite the fact that the national "standard of care" was not available to the participants. The results were impressive: a 50% reduction in neonatal mortality caused by sepsis *(54)*. The benefits of the study for the local people in terms of improved neonatal survival and its impact on national and global programmes for neonatal care have been enormous.

An extreme position on standard of care would have required a control arm that received neonatal intensive care and expensive intravenous antibiotics, neither of which are sustainable even in urban settings in India. Thus, the study could not have taken place and an opportunity for gaining knowledge to reduce neonatal mortality would have been lost.

Another example of a multi-country typhoid vaccine research project details the systematic application of fundamental clinical practice and ethical principles in a developing world public health setting (see Box 1.5). In general, the Good Clinical Practice (GCP) principles are applicable to vaccine trials in developing countries. But they pose complex ethical and practical challenges. In this study, the GCP standards fall into three categories: clearly applicable as stated, clearly applicable as stated but interpretation and application differs between developing and developed countries, and applicable as stated but requires capacity building. The experience from this project potentially contributes to expediting broader access to a well-proven effective vaccine, and may assist the application of new vaccines for the poorest countries in future.

To sum up, the key challenge is how to effectively manage the "global standard" and "local context" interface. This appears to be a universal issue in the ethics of research in developing countries and a process should be developed for resolving it.

Box 1.5 Implementing good clinical practice guidelines in developing countries

The Good Clinical Practice (GCP) principles proposed by the International Conference on Harmonisation of Technical Requirements for Registration of Pharmaceuticals for Human Use provide a standard for the conduct of clinical trials. The aim of GCP is to ensure that the rights, safety and well-being of people participating in such trials are protected and that clinical data are credible and reliable. However, application of these principles in least developed countries (LDCs) poses complex ethical and practical challenges and may require some adaptation to local conditions.

The table below illustrates the implementation of some of the GCP guidelines in LDCs using practical examples from a multi-country typhoid fever vaccine effectiveness trial. In general, the 13 GCP principles are fully applicable to vaccine trials in LDCs, but implementing them falls into three categories: (A) clearly applicable as stated; (B) clearly applicable as stated, but interpretation and application differs between LDCs and developed countries, and (C) applicable as stated, but requires capacity building. Eight out of the 13 GCP principles have been selected as illustrative examples.

Recording information from trial participants in Karachi, Pakistan

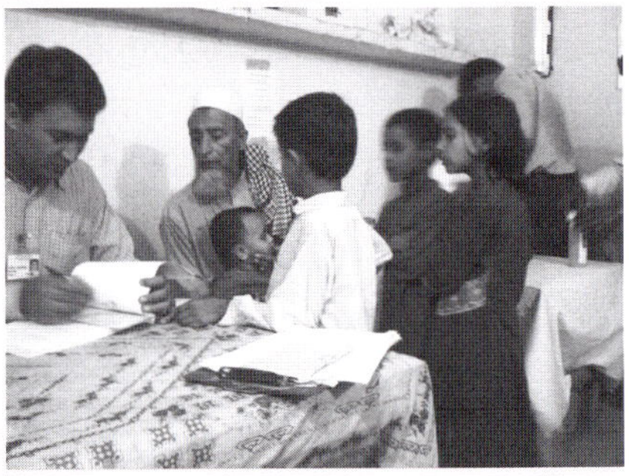

Photo supplied by Dr L Ochiai, International Vaccine Institute, Seoul, Korea.

	Principle	*Applicability **	*Comment*
1.	Clinical trials should be conducted in accordance with ethical principles that originated in the Declaration of Helsinki and are consistent with GCP and applicable regulatory requirement(s).	B	Ethical principles of respect, beneficence, and justice are universal. Major challenge in LDCs because of "vulnerable" study subjects. Distributive justice depends on local assessments. Regulatory requirements may vary considerably or be non-existent.
2.	Before a trial is initiated, foreseeable risks and inconveniences should be weighed against the anticipated benefit for the individual trial participant and society; a trial should be initiated and continued only if the benefits justify the risks.	B	The risk-benefit equation may differ depending on how the investigators and local authorities interpret the available evidence and their local scenario.
3.	The rights, safety and well-being of the trial participants are the most important consideration and should prevail over interests of science and society.	B	Benefits to society could be more relevant in LDCs. In LDCs, herd immunity should be evaluated. In the case of effectiveness trials of licensed vaccines, the vaccine can be offered to the control arm at the end of the project.
6.	A trial should be conducted in compliance with the protocol that has received prior approval or favourable opinion by an ethics committee.	C	In LDCs, local approval and an institutional review of participating organizations should be assured. If local ethics review boards are weak, international review should be sought. Strong commitment to capacity building should be present during the trial.
7.	The medical care given to, and medical decisions made on behalf of, participants should be the responsibility of a qualified physician.	C	LDCs tend to have lower levels of training and experience of professionals. Commitment to capacity and infrastructure building needed. Differences in standards of care should be agreed to in early stages of design.
9.	Freely given informed consent should be obtained from every participant prior to clinical trial participation.	A	Adequate explanation of the research, voluntary consent and suitable documentation are common to developed countries and LDCs. Differences include literacy issues, communal versus individual consent, and level of understanding of technical concepts (randomization, placebo).
11.	Records that could identify participants should be protected, respecting the privacy and confidentiality rules in accordance with the applicable regulatory requirements.	C	In LDCs, names associated with medical and/or socio-demographic information may constitute a threat. Trial participant should be told what precautions would be in place to protect confidentiality as well as any limitations of these.
13.	Systems with procedures that ensure the quality of every aspect of the trial should be implemented.	C	In LDCs an exhaustive approach to ensuring and monitoring quality is not typical in clinical studies. Substantial commitment to capacity building needed.

* A: clearly applicable as stated; B: clearly applicable as stated, but interpretation and application may differ in LDCs and developing countries; C: clearly applicable as stated, but implementation of this guideline requires commitment to capacity building.

Source: Acosta C et al. Implementation of good clinical practice guidelines in vaccine trials in developing countries. a multi-country typhoid fever Vi polysaccharide vaccine evaluation experience. *British Medical Journal*, 2004, in press.

1.6 The process: how was this report developed?

A draft annotated outline of *Knowledge for Better Health* was developed and posted on the Internet in 2003, inviting comments and suggestions. Based on this outline, chapters on key topics in health research were originally commissioned to form the foundation of the report. To help inform the report further, a series of consultations were held in 2004 with researchers, health policy-makers, nongovernmental organizations (NGOs) and donors, such as governments and foundations. It included the formation of two Task Forces: one on Health Systems Research Priorities *(55)* and the other on Knowledge Access and Sharing (38). It also included consultations in all WHO regions* on the broad contents of the report and priorities for research into health systems. Meetings to obtain input from NGOs and government policy-makers were also held.** A consultation to define research priorities in human resources for health also provided input.** The broad consultation process to identify gaps in the research agenda and identify important research questions is still going on.

Seven regional perspectives on priorities for health systems research identified during the regional consultations are highlighted below and again in shaded boxes in the relevant sections of the report:

- **Regional perspective 1:** Priority setting should occur mainly at sub-national (district), national or regional levels rather than at the global level. However, broad, global level priorities were deemed helpful for advocacy and for raising the visibility of health systems research (see Section 2.3)
- **Regional perspective 2:** There is a major need for reliable and timely information on basic indicators pertaining to health systems. This requirement for health systems "benchmarks" was deemed crucial to monitoring and evaluating the achievement of the MDGs, and the performance of the system itself. Included in this is the need for research to develop benchmark indicators for human rights, ethics and equity (see Section 2.3).
- **Regional perspective 3:** A major priority for health systems research should be research into the development of policies for scaling up health services to meet contemporary health challenges (e.g. achieving the MDGs). It should include research on how to better integrate "vertical", single-disease programmes within the broader health system (see Section 2.3).
- **Regional perspective 4:** Further research is needed on regulatory aspects,

* Bangkok, Thailand (March 27–29, 2004); Cairo, Egypt (April 4–6, 2004); Brazzaville, Congo (April 14–16, 2004); Copenhagen, Denmark (April 30, 2004); Mexico City, Mexico (May 24–26, 2004).

** NGOs: Durban, South Africa (June 12, 2004); government policy-makers: Kuala Lumpur, Malaysia (September 16–17, 2004); human resources for health: Cape Town, South Africa, (September 6–8, 2004).

Table 1.2 Suggested topics for health systems research and their potential to affect MDGs

	1	4	5	6	7	8
Financial and human resources						
Community financing and national health insurance	✔	✔	✔	✔		✔
Human resources for health at the district level and below	✔	✔	✔	✔		
Human resource requirements at higher management levels	✔	✔	✔	✔		
Organization and delivery of health services						
Community involvement	✔	✔	✔	✔	✔	
Equitable, effective and efficient health care	✔	✔	✔	✔		
Approaches to the organization of health services	✔	✔	✔	✔		
Drug and diagnostic policies	✔	✔	✔	✔		✔
Governance, stewardship and knowledge management						
Governance and accountability	✔	✔	✔	✔	✔	
Health information systems	✔	✔	✔	✔	✔	
Priority setting and evidence-informed policy making	✔	✔	✔	✔	✔	
Effective approaches for intersectoral engagement in health	✔	✔	✔	✔	✔	✔
Global influences						
Effects of global initiatives and policies (including trade, donors, international agencies) on health systems	✔	✔	✔	✔	✔	✔

✔ = Improved knowledge from health systems research could contribute to attainment of one or more of the targets for the MDG. The relationships are complex and the list is not exhaustive, because attainment of MDGs will be affected by a range of factors interacting both directly and indirectly with health. For example, improved health could contribute to reduction of poverty (MDG 1) through several mechanisms, including reducing loss of income from ill-health and catastrophic expenditures due to illness; and improvements in the health of women and girls could reduce gender disparities in education (MDG 3).

The MDGs in summary

Goal 1: Eradicate extreme poverty and hunger
Goal 2: Achieve universal primary education
Goal 3: Promote gender equality and empower women
Goal 4: Reduce child mortality
Goal 5: Improve maternal health
Goal 6: Combat HIV/AIDS, malaria, and other diseases
Goal 7: Ensure environmental sustainability
Goal 8: Develop a global partnership for development

Source: Task Force on Health Systems Research. Informed choices for attaining the Millennium Development Goals: towards an international cooperative agenda for health systems research. *Lancet*, 2004, 364:997–1003.

corruption and poor governance within health systems in resource-poor countries (see Section 2.3).

- **Regional perspective 5:** Research into ways to improve knowledge transfer and access in health systems should be a priority—it should address the major barriers of financial constraints, language skills, low quality scientific publications at the national and regional levels, and poor access to the Internet (see Section 3.6).

- **Regional perspective 6:** A strong emphasis should be given to improving the linkages between researchers and policy-makers, including the need for developing a cadre of knowledge "brokers" and intermediaries to support national decision-making (see Section 4.5).

- **Regional perspective 7:** Research on how to improve community and

Table 1.3 Research priorities in noncommunicable diseases

Research theme	*Main research questions and information needs*
Burden of disease	■ Age/sex specific death rates by cause, trends over time. ■ Age/sex specific burden of disease rates by cause, trends over time. ■ Better understanding of the potential of prevention (calculation of years of preventable life lost, and what might be achieved through interventions).
Risk factors	■ Standard data on risk factor prevalence by socioeconomic group; trends over time. ■ Life course research on accumulated influences over a lifetime. ■ Socioeconomic inequalities in risk between individuals and regions. ■ Impact of globalization on NCD risk factor prevalence, and trends over time. ■ Increased understanding of determinants of risk factor prevalence.
Diseases and health systems	■ Cost-effective strategies for early detection in low- and middle-income countries. ■ Audit appropriateness and implementation of guidelines and systematic reviews in main NCD areas. ■ Organization of knowledge and information into useful forms for various constituencies. ■ Operational resources to ensure effective treatments reach those in most need. ■ Cost-effectiveness analysis of interventions in different settings. ■ Effective incorporation of prevention strategies into health systems to reach different groups. ■ Develop effective self-management approaches for chronic diseases. ■ Interaction between biologic risk (human genome) and environmental hazards (risk behaviours).
Surveillance	■ Develop core data sets for key risk factors, diseases and mortality. ■ Better use of surveillance to inform health policy. ■ Training in use of surveillance data to monitor progress in prevention, control and research.
Upstream policies	■ Analysis of non health effects (cost of illness, economic effects on families, societies, communities, health services). ■ Research and evaluation on effectiveness and impact of policies, programmes and interventions on health outcomes. ■ Cost effectiveness of health promotion and preventive interventions. ■ Understanding the spread of NCD epidemics to poor populations and appropriate policy responses. ■ Applying new research methods to underlying social, economic, and cultural determinants of NCDs. ■ Balancing spending between communicable diseases and NCDs. ■ Effects of preventive strategies on equity. ■ Research to understand inter-sectoral dynamics in order to advance NCD control (transport, agriculture, financial, social welfare sectors etc). ■ Research on the impact of global and national marketing and pricing policies on diet and nutrition, especially in young people. ■ Investigation of policy drivers to ensure due attention to NCDs. ■ Efforts to increase interdisciplinary research to prevent NCDs. ■ Better understanding of the diffusion of NCD prevention programmes in both developed and developing countries.

NCD: noncommunicable disease

Sources:

(1) *Noncommunicable disease research partners meeting report,* Geneva, World Health Organization, 2002.

(2) Beaglehole R, Chronic diseases: research and policy priorities. In: *The Global Forum Update on Research for Health 2005*, Geneva, Global Forum for Health Research, 2004, in press.

(3) Inputs from M Eriksen, Georgia State University, USA.

grassroots participation in health systems research should be given high priority (see Section 4.6).

These consultations used as their starting point the first draft of a list of 12 priority topics for research to strengthen health systems in low- and middle-income countries developed by the Task Force on Health Systems Research Priorities (see Table 1.2) *(55)*. The broader relevance of these topics is shown by the fact that, for example, effective strategies to promote quality of care generally are also relevant to the development of effective management programmes for noncommunicable diseases (see Table 1.3).

1.7 REORIENTING HEALTH RESEARCH TO STRENGTHEN HEALTH SYSTEMS

"Public health is the art and science of preventing disease, promoting health, and extending life through the organized efforts of society"
(Sir Donald Acheson)

Health research should and can be reoriented to strengthen health systems. To this end, the previous section's review of the current state of global health research reveals three critical areas that need attention: more investment in new approaches to health systems research, better management of critical areas in the health research process, and improved translation of knowledge into actions. The ultimate objective is to facilitate the development of a culture of learning, problem solving and innovation to strengthen health systems, improve health outcomes and equity (see Box 1.6), and build public confidence in science and scientists.

MORE INVESTMENTS IN HEALTH SYSTEMS RESEARCH

Health systems are at the heart of the problem. Health systems research, however, despite acknowledgement of its importance, remains a neglected area that has suffered from under-investment compared to biomedical research. The field often fails to register among major health research priorities at both a national and global level. Research output in this field of research has been miniscule compared to total health and medical research output. In order to generate more support and investment for health systems research there is an urgent need to clearly define where the research gaps and priorities are, and to develop innovative approaches and methodologies. These issues are addressed in **Chapter 2**.

Box 1.6 Promoting health equity

Few countries have proactive, evidence-based national policies aimed at tackling health inequalities head-on. The countries that have tried to reduce inequities include Chile, Mexico, the Netherlands, New Zealand, Sweden, and the United Kingdom. Two analyses have identified at least three common factors that are vital for informing policy to combat health disparities:

- Politicians can use scientific evidence to keep the issue of health inequalities in the public eye and to push health equity up the public agenda. If there is no data on the social distribution of health, the problems remain invisible. It is crucial to present this scientific evidence in non-technical language with illustrative examples to encourage its use as a powerful tool for advocacy.
- Policy-makers, scientists, health professionals, NGOs and the public can join forces to put health inequalities on the public agenda. The research community can provide them with the relevant scientific evidence needed for equity-oriented strategies. It is up to policy-makers and health professionals to ensure these strategies are implemented. It is vital to reach an evidence-based strategy through a democratic process, that is, through dialogue with those who will be affected by the strategy and those who will be responsible for its implementation.
- Health equity is often high on the policy agenda in countries where the government takes international commitments to human justice seriously.

Sources:

Whitehead M. Diffusion of ideas on social inequalities in health: a European perspective. *Milbank Quarterly,* 1998, 76:469–492.

Machenbach JP, Bakker MJ. Tackling socioeconomic inequalities in health: analysis of European experiences. *Lancet,* 2003, 362: 1409–1414.

More effective management of the health research process

Health systems research should be conducted within the broader context of health research in a national setting. **Chapter 3** describes the goals, functions and characteristics of a health research system. All countries need a functioning health research system; each country needs to have the capacity to respond to its own health needs. There is no end point in health where all is known and no more research is needed. There is only a continuous cycle of research, application and evaluation, and learning from that experience.

Where does this learning occur? One of the key contributions of research to health systems is the translation of knowledge into actions—using research to shape health policies, health practices and public opinion. It is in this environment that such learning and problem solving can, and should, occur. The main features of such a learning environment are described in **Chapter 4**. Beyond learning and problem solving, the osmosis of knowledge between the health system and the health research systems should lead, ultimately, to a capacity for innovation in health improvement, based on a willingness to reach beyond traditional academic boundaries to search for cross-fertilizing concepts, approaches and methodologies.

Where do we go from here?

Chapter 5 concludes the report. It presents recommendations and an agenda for action at both national and global level. In the context of the conclusions outlined in the report, what are the challenges and outlook for the future?

The future should ideally be one where there is public trust, confidence and support for health research; where research and evidence inform decisions made by policy-makers, health practitioners and the public; where research helps to narrow the gulf between what it is possible to do and what is actually done; and where the system is responsive to change and unexpected challenges.

How should health research be managed in the future to achieve these goals?

References

1. Bush V. *Science—the endless frontier*. A report to the President by Vannevar Bush, Director of the Office of Scientific Research and Development. Washington, DC, US Government Printing Office, 1945.
2. Callahan D. *What price better health? Hazards of the research imperative*. Berkeley, CA, University of California Press, 2003.
3. Commission on Health Research for Development. *Health research: essential link to equity in development*. Cambridge, MA, Oxford University Press, 1990.
4. Ad Hoc Committee on Health Research Relating to Future Intervention Options. *Investing in Health Research and Development*. Geneva, World Health Organization, 1996.
5. International Organizing Committee. *Report of the International Conference on Health Research for Development, Bangkok, 10–13 October, 2000*. Geneva, 2001.
6. *Health research for development: the continuing challenge*. A discussion paper prepared for the International Conference on Health Research for Development, Bangkok, 10–13 October,

2000 (drafted by MA Lansang, S Tollman, J Kasonde, with support from P Butler). Geneva, Council for Health Research and Development, 2000.
7. Evans T, Whitehead M, Diderichsen F et al. (eds). *Challenging inequities in health: from ethics to action*. New York, Oxford University Press, 2001.
8. Sen G, George A, Ostlin P (eds). *Engendering international health: the challenge of equity*. Cambridge, MA, MIT Press, 2002.
9. Marmot M. *Status syndrome: how your social standing directly affects your health and life expectancy*. London, Bloomsbury, 2004.
10. Labonte L, Schrecker R. *Fatal indifference: The G8, Africa and global health*. Ottawa, International Development Research Centre, 2004.
11. *Genomics and world health*. Geneva, World Health Organization, 2002.
12. Jha P et al. Improving the health of the global poor. *Science*, 2002, 295:2036–2039.
13. Jones G et al. How many child deaths can we prevent this year. *Lancet*, 2003, 362:65–71.
14. Millennium Development Goals (MDGs). http://www.who.int/mdg/en/
15. Wagstaff A, Claeson M. *The Millennium Development Goals for health: rising to the challenges*. Washington, DC, The World Bank, 2004.
16. Travis P et al. Overcoming health-systems constraints to achieve the millennium development goals. *Lancet*, 2004, 364:900–906.
17. Morens DM et al. The challenge of emerging and re-emerging infectious diseases. *Nature*, 2004, 430:242–249.
18. Zimmett P et al. Global and societal implications of the diabetes epidemic. *Nature*, 2001, 414:782–787.
19. *The World Health Report 2000: Health Systems: Improving performance*. Geneva, World Health Organization, 2000.
20. *The World Health Report 2003: Shaping the future*. Geneva, World Health Organization, 2003.
21. Freedman L et al. Millennium project task force 4—child health and maternal health. New York, United Nations Millennium Project, 2004 (accessible at http://www.unmillenniumproject.org/documents/tf4interim.pdf).
22. Pang T et al. Knowledge for better health—a conceptual framework and foundation for health research systems. *Bulletin of the World Health Organization, 2003,* 81:815–820.
23. Garrett L. *Betrayal of trust—the collapse of global public health*. Hyperion, New York, NY, 2000.
24. Wynia M. Professional ethics, broken trust and health disparities. Presentation at 2nd Annual Summer Workshop on Disparities in Health: Working Towards Social Justice. Houston, Texas, July 30, 2004.
25. *The use of genetically modified crops in developing countries*. London, Nuffield Council for Bioethics, 2003.
26. Rymer J et al. Making decisions about hormone replacement therapy. *British Medical Journal*, 2003, 326:322–326.
27. Horton R. The lessons of MMR. *Lancet*, 2004, 363:747–749.
28. Pollack HN. *Uncertain science, uncertain world*. Cambridge, Cambridge University Press, 2003.
29. Phillips B. *The bovine spongiform encephalopathy (BSE) inquiry (The Phillips Inquiry): findings and conclusions*. London, The Stationery Office, 2001.
30. Meldrum M. A "calculated risk": the Salk polio vaccine field trials of 1954. *British Medical Journal*, 1998, 317:1233–1236.
31. Wasi P. *Triangle that moves the mountain and health systems reform movement in Thailand*. Bangkok, Health Systems Research Institute, 2000.
32. *The 10/90 report on health research, 2003–2004*. Geneva, Global Forum for Health Research, 2004.
33. Commission on Macroeconomics and Health. *Macroeconomics and health: investing in health for economic development*. Geneva, World Health Organization, 2001.
34. A manual for research priority setting using the ENHR strategy. Geneva, Council for Health Research and Development, 2000.

35. Ghaffar A, de Francisco A, Matlin S (eds). The combined matrix approach: a priority-setting tool for health research. Geneva, Global Forum for Health Research, 2004.
36. Keiser J et al. Gender composition of editorial boards of general medical journals. *Lancet*, 2003, 362:1336.
37. Horton R. Medical journals: evidence of bias against the diseases of poverty. *Lancet*, 2003, 361:712–713.
38. Godlee F et al. Can we achieve health information for all by 2015? *Lancet*, 2004, 364: 295–300.
39. Egger M, Davey Smith, G, Altmann DG (eds). *Systematic reviews in health care: meta-analysis in context*. London, BMJ Publishing Group, 2nd edition, 2001.
40. Hunt M. *How science takes stock: the story of meta analysis*. New York, NY, Russell Sage Foundation, 1997.
41. Swingler GH, Volmink J, Ioannidis JP. Number of published systematic reviews and global burden of disease: database analysis. *British Medical Journal*, 2003, 327:1083–1084.
42. Chalmers I. Under-reporting research is scientific misconduct. *Journal of the American Medical Association*, 1990, 263:1405–1408.
43. Ramchandani P. A question of balance: how safe are the medicines that are prescribed to children? *Nature*, 2004, 430:401–402.
44. Marshal E. Buried data can be hazardous to a company's health. *Science*, 2004, 304: 1576–1577.
45. Meier B. Group weighs plan for full drug-trial disclosure. *The New York Times*, June 15, 2004.
46. Harris G. New York state official sues drug maker over test data. *The New York Times*, June 3, 2004.
47. Steinbrook R. Public registration of clinical trials. *New England Journal of Medicine*, 2004, 351:315–317.
48. De Angelis C et al. Clinical trial registration: a statement from the international committee of medical journal editors. *New England Journal of Medicine*, 2004, 351:1250–1251.
49. Evans T et al. Registering clinical trials: an essential role for WHO. *Lancet*, 2004, 363: 1413–1414.
50. Dickersin K, Rennie D. Registering clinical trials. *Journal of the American Medical Association*, 2003, 290:516–523.
51. *The ethics of research related to healthcare in developing countries*. London, Nuffield Council on Bioethics, 2002.
52. Emanuel EJ et al. What makes clinical research in developing countries ethical? The benchmarks of ethical research. *Journal of Infectious Diseases*, 2004, 189:930–937.
53. *International ethics guidelines for biomedical research involving human subjects*. Geneva, Council for International Organizations of Medical Sciences, 2002.
54. Bang AT et al. Effect of home-based neonatal care and management of sepsis on neonatal mortality: field trial in rural India. *Lancet*, 1999, 354:1955–1961.
55. Task Force on Health Systems Research. Informed choices for attaining the millennium development goals: towards an international cooperative agenda for health systems research. *Lancet*, 2004, 364:997–1003.

2

Towards a Scientific Basis for Health Systems

"Health systems should nurture a stronger culture of learning and problem-solving to tackle the major health challenges of our times. This could be achieved through a greater understanding of how the diverse elements within a health system interact with each other, and by finding innovative ways to solve complex problems."
(Tim Evans)

Key Messages

- Health systems in the developing world face major problems related to shortages, maldistribution and waste of financial, human, knowledge and other resources, and coverage shortfalls. There is increasing recognition by major health initiatives that many of their efforts to improve health share the same common health system constraints.
- Despite acknowledgement of its importance and potential to overcome health system constraints, health systems research suffers from a poor image and has been neglected and under-funded compared to other areas of health research.
- Key research issues and knowledge gaps pertaining to human resources, financing, health information and delivery of health services must be addressed in the context of more emphasis on broader health systems strengthening.
- Based on a readiness to reach beyond traditional academic disciplines, innovations, new methodologies and better tools should be developed for health systems research.
- A substantial programme to support the

Interesting numbers

1 million	Estimated number of additional health workers needed if the MDGs are to be achieved in sub-Saharan Africa.
2%	Percentage of global health expenditure in Africa, which carries 25% of the global burden of disease. In contrast, 90% of global health spending is in developed countries with 20% of the world's population.
2%	Percentage of countries in WHO's Africa and South-East Asia regions that have complete coverage of death registration data, as opposed to 75% in the European region.
0.71%	Percentage of papers on the subject of health systems and health services research in the year 2000 based on a search of Medline.
0.1%	Percentage allocated to health systems research as a portion of total health expenditure in developing countries.

(Sources for these numbers are given on the report web site: www.who.int/rpc/wr2004)

development of a new paradigm for research to strengthen health systems is required in the near term if health systems are to perform more effectively and improve health outcomes.

2.1 Bottlenecks and constraints in health systems

The major constraints and challenges currently facing health systems in the developing world include: workforce shortages, limited financing, scant or poor quality health information, shortfalls in coverage of essential health services, problems with quality, and inability to scale up rapidly *(1)*. The major constraints in these areas will be elaborated upon in this section.

Human resources

Although most health systems spend the majority of their funds on the health workforce, there is a paradoxical absence of policy or programmatic discourse on this critical resource. Moreover, the workforce has suffered from being regarded as a recurrent cost that is to be minimized, rather than as a valued asset of the system that needs to be enriched. The idea that health systems are unable to function without workers sounds remarkably obvious but the realization that the workforce is critical to saving lives is often taken for granted and/or ignored. Recent evidence (see Figure 2.1) suggests, however, that more health workers can be associated with lower infant, child and maternal mortality.

Despite their importance to health achievement, there is a growing body of evidence pointing to a shortage of about four million health workers globally *(2)*. In sub-Saharan Africa, where this shortage is most pronounced (see

Figure 2.1 Relationship between mortality and health workforce

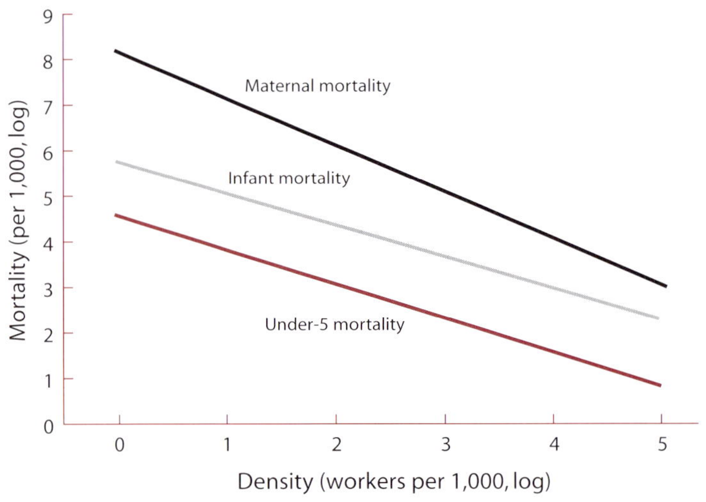

Source: Joint Learning Initiative (JLI) on Human Resources for Health and Development, Strategy Report, September, 2004.

Figure 2.2), it is estimated that an additional one million health workers need to be mobilized if the MDGs are to be achieved. At the same time, countries in the Organisation for Economic Development and Cooperation (OECD), which represents much of the industrialized and developed world, are facing shortages of health workers too, mainly due to an expansion of the health sector. These shortfalls are being met increasingly by workers from poorer countries *(3)*. In countries where health workers are already scarce, increasing migration is associated with the interruption of life-saving services sometimes referred to as "fatal flows" in the health workforce. The migration of health workers also occurs within countries *(4)* where nurses and doctors are lured away from the public sector by higher private sector pay, and the magnet of urban life depletes the workforce in rural areas.

Beyond these shortages, there are a number of factors that prevent health workers from having the best opportunities to improve health and alleviate suffering. Antiquated curricula in medical schools mean that professionals are often ill-equipped to respond to the needs of the population, creating a so-called "skills-gap". The primary employers of health workers including governments, NGOs and the private sector often fail to provide "productive" working conditions. These range from irregular to inadequate pay, an absence of requisite supplies such as drugs and diagnostics, as well as a lack of incentives to encourage workers to serve in remote, isolated locations.

Finally, not enough is known about the demographics of health workers due to an absence of standard definitions for these workers and a lack of methods to accurately assess the size and composition of this workforce. Data on specific cadres such as community health workers or doctors and nurses working in the private sector, and breakdowns of these by gender, tend to be sketchy.

Figure 2.2 Health workforce by region

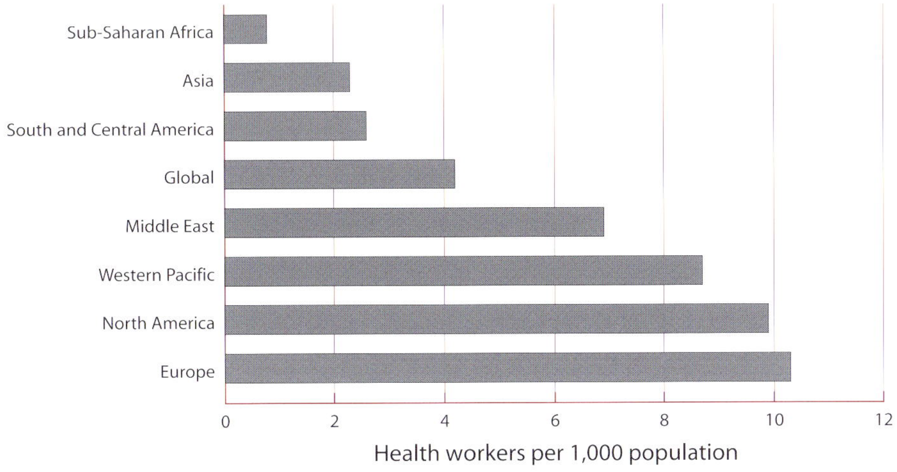

Source: Joint Learning Initiative (JLI) on Human Resources for Health and Development, Strategy Report, September, 2004.

Financing

Not only a massive mobilization of human resources, but also substantial financial resources are needed for the health sector in a number of countries. The debate about achieving the MDGs for health in developing countries has raised questions about how big the health system needs to be to attain those targets. Various estimates within and across countries call for significantly more spending in the health sector. This recognition of the need to expand the health sector in poor countries along with the recent emergence of large international funds has raised fundamental questions as to whether the macroeconomic frameworks that have guided public spending across all social sectors in the past are appropriate for the health sector (5). Moreover, the availability of new funds raises new important issues related to the tracking of expenditures and the understanding of costs and benefits of alternative investments. Furthermore, the provision of treatment through new schemes, for example antiretroviral therapy for people living with HIV/AIDS, raises the issue of how the health system can sustain this expenditure in the long term.

Across most health systems, there is widespread agreement with the principle that a sick individual should be able to receive appropriate care without compromising their own or their family's livelihoods. Unfortunately, people in many countries have access to health care but only at great personal expense and, in many cases, they may be pushed into poverty. High levels of what is known as out-of-pocket payment can lead to financial catastrophe and impoverishment for many households. The proportion of households affected by this varies according to the health system characteristics of a country *(6)* (see Table 2.1). This poses an enormous challenge to develop fair ways of financing the health system. Despite considerable experience with alternative health financing schemes around the world, the prospects for measurable progress on this front are bleak, especially in the weakest economies. Sustainable financing of essential health services for the poor remains a major hurdle and many households struggle to pay for their own health care. One of the top priorities for health systems is to create a fair, long-term scheme to finance health systems. The ultimate goal would be universal coverage.

To help countries meet these challenges, it is important to find ways to routinely obtain information on key financing parameters. This includes information on how much is spent, by whom and for what, and whether households suffer catastrophic financial payments. It also includes information on the costs, effectiveness and implications for equity of using health resources in particular ways, something that is necessary to decide how best to achieve stated health system objectives.

Health information

On his first day of office in an address to staff of WHO, the new Director-General, Dr Lee Jong-wook, described health information as the "glue that holds health systems together". In remarks on the need to strengthen and integrate health information systems at country level, he noted that countries

Table 2.1 Out-of-pocket health payments, catastrophic payments and impoverishment, 59 countries, various years 1991–2000

Country	Share of households with catastrophic health expenditures (%)	Share of households impoverished by out-of-pocket payments for health (%)	Out-of-pocket payment share of total health expenditure (%)
Argentina	5.77	6.7	41.3
Azerbaijan	7.15	4.3	65.7
Bangladesh	1.21	3.4	53.7
Belgium	0.09	0.0	21.8
Brazil	10.27	5.1	61.3
Bulgaria	2.00	3.3	49.8
Cambodia	5.02	2.9	89.7
Canada	0.09	0.0	16.9
Colombia	6.26	3.3	41.5
Costa Rica	0.12	3.0	7.5
Croatia	0.20	1.2	9.5
Czech Republic	0.00	0.0	10.1
Denmark	0.07	0.0	13.7
Djibouti	0.32	1.8	39.2
Egypt	2.80	2.8	79.2
Estonia	0.31	3.7	20.2
Finland	0.44	0.1	25.7
France	0.01	0.1	11.5
Germany	0.03	0.0	10.2
Ghana	1.30	3.6	57.7
Greece	2.17	0.6	46.1
Guyana	0.60	5.1	22.8
Hungary	0.20	0.5	25.3
Iceland	0.30	0.0	20.3
Indonesia	1.26	1.7	76.8
Israel	0.35	0.4	24.0
Jamaica	1.86	5.0	29.3
Kyrgyzstan	0.62	0.4	36.2
Latvia	2.75	3.4	38.4
Lebanon	5.17	3.1	64.4
Lithuania	1.34	2.1	24.0
Mauritius	1.28	1.4	56.4
Mexico	1.54	1.3	43.2
Morocco	0.17	1.8	58.2
Namibia	0.11	1.2	10.8
Nicaragua	2.05	3.6	29.6
Norway	0.28	2.9	15.3
Panama	2.35	0.0	28.5
Paraguay	3.51	2.5	60.3
Peru	3.21	3.7	48.6
Philippines	0.78	2.7	48.5
Portugal	2.71	1.8	37.1
Republic of Korea	1.73	1.8	51.5
Romania	0.09	2.3	17.4
Senegal	0.55	2.0	70.3
Slovakia	0.00	0.1	4.1
Slovenia	0.06	1.6	11.3

continued

Table 2.1 Out-of-pocket health payments, catastrophic payments and impoverishment, 59 countries, various years 1991–2000 *(continued)*

Country	*Share of households with catastrophic health expenditures (%)*	*Share of households impoverished by out-of-pocket payments for health (%)*	*Out-of-pocket payment share of total health expenditure (%)*
South Africa	0.03	1.3	9.7
Spain	0.48	0.4	19.0
Sri Lanka	1.25	3.5	59.2
Sweden	0.18	0.3	19.0
Switzerland	0.57	0.1	16.8
Thailand	0.80	1.5	40.4
Ukraine	3.87	4.0	38.9
United Kingdom	0.04	0.2	4.6
United States of America	0.55	0.4	22.9
Viet Nam	10.45	7.7	80.8
Yemen	1.66	2.7	50.6
Zambia	2.29	1.9	47.8

Source: all variables estimated from households survey data, various years 1991–2000.

Reference: Xu K, Evans DB, Kawabata K, et al. Household catastrophic health expenditure: a multi-country analysis. *Lancet*, 2003, 362:111–117.

with the highest disease burden are the least likely to count births and deaths, and he concluded that "to make people count, we first need to be able to count people". The "gold standard" of national registration systems currently covers only one third of estimated global mortality *(1)*. Many countries cannot even count their dead (see Table 2.2).

As major initiatives get underway, such as the MDGs and the 3 by 5 strategy to provide antiretroviral therapy to 3 million people with HIV/AIDS by 2005, more information is needed on how to implement these programmes in developing countries. The many international and uncoordinated efforts to obtain this information represent the "perfect storm" that jeopardizes already fragile information systems in many developing countries *(7)*. This is both a threat and an opportunity. From the potential destruction wrought by the storm rises an opportunity to reform and strengthen information systems. All key stakeholders must join forces to construct a robust platform through which quality information can flow in a more sustainable manner *(7)*.

The aim of the health information system is to collect, process, report and use health information and knowledge to influence policy-making, programme

Table 2.2 Availability of death registration data in WHO Regions

Region	*Usable data*	*Complete coverage*	*Total countries*
Africa	4	1	46
Americas	32	14	35
South-East Asia	4	0	11
Europe	48	39	51
Eastern Mediterranean	7	4	22
Western Pacific	22	8	27
Total	117	66	192

Source: World Health Report 2003, World Health Organization.

action and research. In practice, country health information systems lack cohesion, having developed in a piecemeal way, fashioned by administrative, economic, legal or donor pressures. Responsibility for health information is sometimes spread across different ministries or institutions within a country. Special efforts are needed to ensure that the distribution of this information is coordinated properly and shared with the health sector.

Ministries and institutions, however, often resist coordinating this due to financial and administrative constraints. Counting births and deaths—a basic building block of the health information system—is generally the task of planning or interior ministries, rather than ministries of health.

Household surveys containing a wealth of health-related data are often carried out by national statistics offices and their links with health ministries are often weak. Data generated through the routine activities of health facilities, such as hospitals or clinics, may not be taken into consideration because this may be seen as being of low quality and having poor coverage. Moreover, in some countries the burgeoning private sector is often poorly regulated and does not provide essential data to the health authorities.

Into this already complex picture come new challenges to health systems and to health information systems. In the context of health sector reform and of decentralization, health systems are managed as closely to the population as possible, often at district level, in order to be more responsive to the needs of the people. This shift in functions between the central and peripheral levels generates new information needs and calls for an in-depth restructuring of information systems, with new requirements for collecting, processing, analysing and disseminating data. Interim reports on a wide range of health criteria as part of efforts to attain the MDGs to improve health in developing countries have exposed the weakness of country health information systems.

Health services delivery

The human, financial, information, and technical/material resources of a health system merge to provide health services. At present, this "merging" or in other words these "health services" fall far short of performance expectations of important health outcomes. Not only are populations in greatest need not receiving tried and tested treatment and medicines, but many health problems remain invisible. People who turn to the system for health care, sometimes at great personal expense, often fail to receive intended health benefits. This disappointing performance of the health system is of great concern and requires a more fundamental understanding of its complex determinants.

In many developing countries, the major health system constraint is the inability to rapidly scale up activities to meet contemporary health challenges. This is directly related to the broader issue of the organization of health services delivery and the tension that exists between single disease or vertical programme approaches and a more holistic approach to health-care delivery.

Ensuring equitable, universal access to health care—whether preventive, promotive or curative—is a key objective of health systems. Key constraints in achieving this relate to low levels of coverage for many priority interventions, poor coordination and weak infrastructure. Conflicting agendas of donor programmes and diversion of trained workers into high-profile initiatives compound the problem in developing countries.

Constraints in the context of MDGs

Efforts to achieve the MDGs pose special challenges to overburdened health systems. Table 2.3 lists the challenges and barriers to improving health service delivery identified in reviews of major health initiatives that attempt to make treatments for diseases like AIDS, tuberculosis and malaria—as well as vaccines and health information—more widely available *(8)*. The table shows shortages of skilled health workers, lack of funds, shortages of medicines, inability to generate and use information, and inadequate public health information systems. Reviews of other programmes and initiatives dealing with noncommunicable diseases and injuries, for example, face similar systems constraints.

Current constraints facing health systems must therefore be seen beyond the lens of one specific health problem and more in the context of a need to consider broader health systems strengthening. There are increasing concerns that a singular emphasis on "vertical", that is single-disease or single-intervention, programmes may no longer be adequate to deal with the entire spectrum of today's global health challenges. The discourse involving major global health initiatives, such as Stop TB and 3 by 5, emphasizes their need to take into consideration the broader health system context, and to contribute to overall system strengthening *(8)*. The increasing burden of noncommunicable diseases in the developing world, such as obesity, diabetes and cardiovascular disease, also underscores the need for broader, more comprehensive systems that are able to deal with the challenges of providing continuous care.

In recognition of this shift, broader health systems strengthening is a core principle of 3 by 5. To help developing countries achieve this goal, WHO has set up an HIV/AIDS and Health Systems Platform to complement other efforts in those countries to improve HIV/AIDS prevention and treatment.

This shift in emphasis to a more holistic approach poses some challenges for health services delivery as well as systems monitoring (see Section 2.4).

2.2 Health systems research

Given the enormous challenges facing health systems today, a robust and sound research enterprise is critical in generating the knowledge needed to overcome these constraints. This area of research is referred to as health systems research.

What is health systems research?

Health systems research is defined as the generation and utilization of new knowledge to improve the way societies achieve their health goals. This may include the way they plan, manage and finance efforts to improve health, as

Table 2.3 Barriers and challenges to improving service delivery identified in reviews of major initiatives

	Maternal health	*Child health*	*TB*	*Malaria*	*HIV/AIDS*
Community and household level					
Demand-side barriers—individual: socioeconomic, gender effects on behaviour, access, use of care	✔	✔	✔	✔	✔
Demand-side barriers—community: absence of social pressures to improve access	✔		✔		✔
Stigma*	✔		✔		✔
Health services delivery					
Inequitable availability of services	✔	✔	✔	✔	✔
Multiple providers, public and private	✔	✔	✔	✔	✔
Provider behaviour to clients	✔	✔	✔	✔	✔
Case management: poor adherence, increasing drug resistance, adverse events	✔	✔	✔	✔	✔
Physical infrastructure, equipment	✔	✔	✔	✔	✔
Human resources availability and management, including payment mechanisms, quality of care, supervision	✔	✔	✔	✔	✔
Drug supplies, supply systems	✔	✔	✔	✔	✔
Service management capacity	✔	✔	✔	✔	✔
Referral and other communication failures	✔	✔	✔		
Health sector policy, strategic management					
High level political commitment to the specific problem or programme	✔	✔	✔		✔
Financial constraints, resource allocation	✔	✔	✔	✔	✔
Insufficient coordination between donors, non-governmental organisations, government bodies	✔	✔	✔	✔	✔
Regulation or legislation to affect both public and private actors	✔	✔	✔	✔	✔
Weak links between programmes leading to inefficiencies and competition for limited resources	✔	✔	✔	✔	
Sector-wide approaches, health-sector reforms	✔		✔		
Monitoring systems, use of information—public and private sector	✔	✔	✔	✔	✔
Public policies cutting across sectors					
Macroeconomic policies, poverty reduction strategies, civil service rules and reforms	✔	✔	✔		

TB = Tuberculosis

✔ Indicates challenge or barrier faced by that health priority

* Although stigma is not always perceived as a health-system issue, it is included here because health systems can reduce or increase stigma, depending on the way people are treated by providers and perhaps the availability of effective treatment.

Source: Travis P et al. Overcoming health systems constraints to achieve the Millennium Development Goals, *Lancet*, 2004, 364:900–906.

well as involving and engaging all interested sectors of society *(9)*. Health systems research is essentially research that investigates strategies for improving health service delivery, including the use of sound evidence in developing such strategies and in shaping effective health policy. It may be applied both within institutions, communities and at district or national level.

Taking stock of health systems research

The need for more support and commitment to health systems research is not a new idea. The European Commission has been supporting health systems and policy research in developing countries through its International Scientific Cooperation programme, which was established in 1983 and is now known as INCO. These efforts have focused on socioeconomic factors, research for policy decisions, health care services intervention and research to action in reproductive health. WHO has been promoting the importance of health systems research for nearly 40 years *(10)* and had a dedicated Health Systems Research and Development Programme from 1989–1998 within its Division for Strengthening of Health Services. In the late 1980s, WHO even considered establishing a Special Programme on Health Systems Research and Development, following the model of Special Programmes on Tropical Disease Research (TDR) and Human Reproduction Research (HRP). Both TDR and HRP have also included health systems research in their portfolio of activities, especially those related to capacity building in countries.

The International Health Policy Programme (IHPP) was established between 1986 and 1998 and focused on establishing teams of researchers and policy-makers in developing countries *(11)*.The World Health Assembly in 1990 recommended that WHO should integrate rather than compartmentalize health systems research and that "such an approach should include the appropriate components of WHO special programmes, national capacity building efforts, and an international health policy programme" *(10)*. In 1996, a WHO report articulated a research agenda for health policy and systems development *(12)* addressing central issues of financing, public/private mix, decentralization, quality of health services and monitoring systems, among others. More recently, the Alliance for Health Policy and Systems Research (AHPSR), an initiative of the Global Forum for Health Research, was launched in 2000 to promote the generation, dissemination and use of knowledge for enhancing health system performance.

Why has health systems research had a limited impact?

Why, despite these activities, and continuous acknowledgement of its importance, has progress in health systems research been slow?

As mentioned in Chapter 1, health systems research has traditionally been underfunded and relatively neglected compared to health and medical research in general. Also, it has largely failed to benefit from increases in investment in recent years for research into diseases of poverty. According to the most recent 10/90 Report on Health Research (2003–2004) *(13)*, health systems research attracts less than one tenth of 1% of total health expenditure in low-income countries. Within the US National Institutes of Health, it has been estimated that less than 2% of the total research budget is allocated for health services research *(14)*. In 1991, health services research accounted for only 0.27% of articles cited in Medline *(9)*. This had increased to 0.71% in 2000 but still represents a fraction of the total. Most of these articles were studies conducted in the developed world.

Health systems research has not always been successful in attracting the best minds, and seems unable to compete with scientific disciplines such as biomedical and clinical research which are seen as more glamorous and high-profile. Similarly, career prospects and advancement within academia seemed more limited for those choosing this career path. In large organizations dealing with health, such as ministries of health and WHO, administrative structures are often not conducive for allowing health systems research to flourish. Table 2.4 lists some of the possible reasons for this relative neglect including poor image, long timeframes, methodological constraints, context-specificity and inability to generalize, and difficulty in assessing the impact of the research *(8)*.

As a scientific discipline, health systems research has not been successful in developing a frontier or cutting-edge image and has, at the same time, also had difficulty in bridging its more fundamental components with the more applied, problem-solving objectives. Importantly, health systems research has had difficulty in shaking off the image of being a diffuse and "fluffy" area of scientific research that is often perceived as lacking a sharp focus and direction. However, it is not all gloom, and two examples of health systems research that have had an impact at district and national levels are provided. In the context of health sector reform and decentralization in Tanzania, community-based participatory research conducted by the Tanzania Essential Health Interven-

Table 2.4 Some reasons for neglect of health systems research

- **Health systems have an image problem**: visible or emotive topics such as child deaths or polio campaigns engage stakeholders in ways that interventions for strengthening planning or accountability mechanisms do not.
- **Health systems research also has an image problem**: other forms of research such as basic science and drug discovery are prestigious while health systems research is seen as fluffy, pedestrian and applied. This attitude is caused by divergent views on the types of systems issues that can be researched, and to methodological challenges.
- **Divergent views on the types of questions amenable to scientific enquiry**: some believe that health system problems are primarily political, and therefore best solved using common sense rather than evidence.
- **Answers from such research can be slow to arrive and uncertain**, because of the long-term nature of health systems change, and the complex and indirect links to final outcomes.
- **Generalization can be difficult,** because the effects of interventions crucially depend on the environment in which they are implemented.
- **Health systems research may not have a disease-specific or intervention-specific focus**, so there are fewer research opportunities for research funding.
- **Disinterest and difficulty in assessment:** because the interventions are part of large messy reforms with strong political imperatives; systematic evaluations are difficult to design and may be difficult to defend.
- **Restricted research capacity, and a research workforce that is multi-disciplinary** and therefore does not have an obvious institutional home with clear career structures.
- **The right questions are not being asked**: improved understanding is needed about the types of research that really changes the way decision-makers think.

Source: Travis P et al. Overcoming health systems constraints to achieve the Millennium Development Goals, *Lancet*, 2004, 364: 900–906.

tions Project (TEHIP) resulted in a better match between disease burden and resource allocation at the district level (see Box 2.1). In Laos, rapid economic reforms led to a major problem with substandard and fake drugs on the market. Research performed by Lao and Swedish researchers in the area of access and quality of medicines was directly responsible for the adoption of a national drug policy in 1993, which was passed into law in 2000 (see Box 2.2).

The following section offers a potentially more targeted approach to health systems research by identifying knowledge gaps in the four core dimensions of health system performance where research can make an impact: human resources, financing, information and delivery of services.* The work of the Task Force on Health Systems Research Priorities (see Section 1.6) also identified 12 priority topics for health systems research *(15)*.

2.3 WHAT ARE THE KNOWLEDGE GAPS IN HEALTH SYSTEMS?

Although health systems research cannot be expected to solve all of the problems facing health systems, it does have a central role to play. However, the priority research questions need to be identified and addressed in order to improve the knowledge base. Such topics may focus on noncommunicable diseases or on efforts underway to achieve the MDGs, but it is just as important to conduct research on the way a health system functions. Based on the health system constraints identified in a previous section, the knowledge gaps and research priorities in key health system functions will be described.

Regional perspective 1

Priority setting should occur mainly at sub-national (district), national or regional levels rather than at the global level. However, broad, global level priorities were deemed helpful for advocacy and for raising the visibility of health systems research.

HUMAN RESOURCES

A more solid knowledge and evidence base would help to inform the challenges associated with the health workforce. A recent priority setting workshop in human resources for health (HRH) research proposed that research should be organized around seven key themes *(2)*:

1. Assessment, policy and planning
2. Managing size, skill mix and organization
3. Using incentives to improve performance

* Another key dimension of health systems is stewardship *(18)*. Although this is not analysed in any great depth in this report, stewardship can be considered as an overarching function which guides human resources, financing, information and delivery of services. It should be mentioned, however, that it may, in and of itself, contain some knowledge gaps relating to public/private mix, managing change etc.

Box 2.1 How Tanzania is using research to reform its health system

The Tanzania Essential Health Interventions Project (TEHIP) was set up to find new ways to plan, set priorities and allocate resources as part of a major reform of the country's health-care system. Tanzanian researchers started research in 1997 in two of the country's 123 districts—Rufiji and Morogoro—as part of the project run by the Ministry of Health and Canada's International Development Research Centre. Latest data from a five-year follow-up of the project indicate a 54% reduction in infant mortality, a 47% reduction in under-five mortality and a 18% reduction in adult mortality.

The research project is focused on health systems, health behaviours, health impacts, and the research and development of planning tools. The initial aim was to evaluate the overall impact of health interventions in terms of burdens of disease and per capita cost. For example, the researchers found that in both Rufiji and Morogoro districts, malaria alone accounted for 30% of all healthy years of life lost due to deaths in 1996–1997. In response, government planners increased the budget for malaria prevention and treatment programmes from just 10% to 26% by 2000–2001 (see figure). The research also showed that children under five carried more than 60% of the total burden of disease in both districts, compared with 37% for adults.

Overall, the research has resulted in a better match between disease burden and health budget allocation (see figure). It also helped to develop tools to help district health management teams collect and analyse information, improve health service delivery, set priorities and allocate resources accordingly.

Burden of Disease Profiles draw from sentinel demographic surveillance areas to show health needs at the community level. District Health Accounts map district health budgets and expenditures in relation to the burden of disease and other criteria. The third tool, the Integrated Management Cascade, is a hierarchical communications and supervisory support structure that delegates responsibilities within the health system. The fourth is the Community Driven Facility Rehabilitation, which aims to improve health service delivery, community responsibility and involvement.

Using these four tools, Rufiji and Morogoro districts have addressed their burden of disease by investing in several essential health interventions, such as the Integrated Management of Childhood Illnesses strategy, insecticide-treated bednets and the Safe Motherhood Initiative. By redirecting health spending using TEHIP's tools, both districts have cut their child mortality rate by more than 40% since the late 1990s.

Tanzania has initiated similar per capita health funding in at least two thirds of the country through a new, sector-wide government-donor partnership. To promote this evidence-based approach to health-care funding, TEHIP has printed manuals in English and Swahili and developed training courses with the Ministry of Health.

The government has started to introduce the cascade method to other districts and is poised to do the same with the facility rehabilitation tool as well. It is training officials in districts to use the tools that can help match a region's burden of disease profile with a corresponding budget. The goal is to have all the districts using these tools to allocate resources according to health priorities by the 2005 planning cycle.

Fixing Health Systems, *published by the International Development Research Centre, Ottawa, Canada, in October 2004, and other resources on the project, are available at www.idrc.ca/tehip.*

A better match between budget allocation and disease burden: health expenditures in Morogoro district 1996–97 and 2000–01

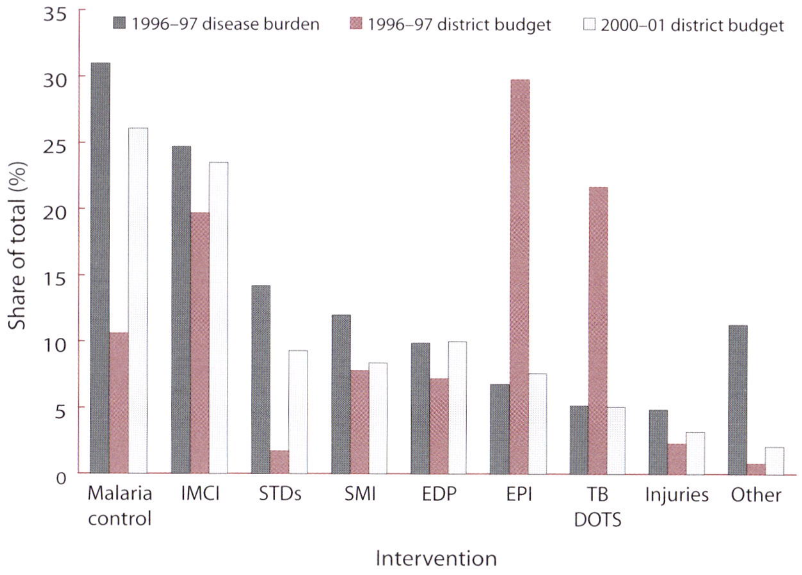

Legend

IMCI: Integrated Management of Childhood Illness
STDs: Sexually Transmitted Diseases
SMI: Severe Mental Illness
EDP: Essential Drug Programme
EPI: Extended Programme on Immunization
TB DOTS: Tuberculosis Directly Observed Treatment, Short Course Strategy

4. Mobility
5. Educating and training
6. Legislation and regulation
7. Influence of political and macroeconomic contexts on the development of national HRH strategies and policies

Although these themes reasonably capture the scope of issues that are important in the management of the workforce, they do not reveal much about the nature of the research questions and their relative importance. Specifically, across each of these dimensions there is a set of fundamental and empirical

Box 2.2 Lao national drug policy

Economic reform in the Lao People's Democratic Republic in 1987 triggered the explosive growth in the pharmaceutical industry and the arrival of substandard and fake drugs on the market. It became easy to obtain drugs without prescriptions, pharmacy staff were not trained properly, patients overused antibiotics, and consumers were provided with little or no information when they bought medicines.

To tackle these problems, the Lao government—aided by the Swedish International Development and Cooperation Agency (SIDA) and in collaboration with various ministries, provincial health offices, health professional groups, the Lao Women's Union, NGOs, and donor agencies—developed a National Drug Policy (NDP). Launched in 1993, the goals were to:

- reduce the prevalence of substandard and fake drugs
- induce rational use of drugs and use of drugs relevant to the health-care needs of the population
- improve the quality of drug transactions between drug sellers and customers
- implement a quality assessment mechanism.

To improve the chances of the NDP's success, policy-makers adopted a multisectoral approach involving provinces, districts and villages. A stepwise model for capacity building was designed so that, eventually, the programme could run without external assistance. Routine assessment using established indicators was considered of key importance to allow for evidence-based ongoing revision and informed decision-making. Institutional strengthening is promoted through learning experiences such as seminars and health systems research projects.

One other important factor has been the inter-institutional collaboration between a multidisciplinary group at the Division of International Health, Karolinska Institute in Sweden and the Lao Ministry of Health.

Ten years after the NDP was launched, the list of achievements has been impressive:

- During Phase I (1993–1995) a Food and Drug Quality Control Centre was established with trained laboratory staff, 123 inspectors were trained, the essential drug list was revised and the banned drug list elaborated.
- Phase II (1996–2000) brought the Phase I capacity-building activities to action through national implementation as well as boosted pilot implementation in the five major provinces. This involved additional training, technical assistance, equipment, and transport, as well as pharmacy inspections, standard treatment guideline development, and monitoring of rational drug use.
- Evaluation studies during Phase II found drastic improvements in private pharmacy service quality from 1997-1999, provision of drug information to customers rose from 35% to 51% and the presence of substandard drugs dropped from 44% to 22% of random samples.
- Phase III (2001–2003) focused on continuing improvements through routine inspections and self-assessments, developing a self-financing system, and strengthening management capacity.

13 elements of revised Lao NDP, 2001

1. Law and regulation
2. Drug selection
3. Drug nomenclature
4. Quality assurance (registration, licensing, quality surveillance)
5. Drug advertising
6. Drug supply (procurement, distribution, storage)
7. Rational use of drugs
8. Strategy on drug economy
9. Traditional medicine
10. Operational research
11. Organization, management and monitoring of NDP
12. Human resources development
13. Technical cooperation

Source: National Drug Policy Programme, 1993–2003. Ministry of Health, Food and Drug Department, Vientiane, Lao PDR, 2003.
Rolf Wahlstrom and Goran Tomson. Personal communication.

research questions that must be addressed but have yet to register as research priorities. These include such things as: How does one assess the state of the health workforce? What is the optimal skill mix? How many workers are migrating and to where? How many health education institutions are there in a given country or region? Similarly, there is a series of more applied and contextually specific questions that should also register as credible research: How can worker productivity be enhanced in district health centres? What types of recruitment and incentive packages work for attracting and retaining workers in remote areas? How are two tiers of salaries managed among workers in a hospital introducing an AIDS treatment programme?

Financing

Health system financing is a broad area. It covers: inputs such as health expenditure, revenue collection, fund pooling and purchasing, and the measurement of key health system outcomes such as catastrophic health expenditures and impoverishment. Within the financing function, there are important unanswered research questions relating to the three sub-functions: revenue collection, pooling and purchasing, as well as to the interactions between them. Table 2.5 shows one perspective on research priorities for all these areas. Here, a distinction is made between research on inputs, the financing function, and outcome assessment and monitoring. It highlights some areas of contemporary interest including macro-financing issues and community participation in payment of health services and health insurance schemes.

Health information

The results generated by the health information system are needed to guide and complement health research, from the design of research projects to the interpretation of the findings. Conversely, health research can contribute significantly to the rapid enhancement of country information systems by identifying data dissemination strategies that enable information to be shared effectively to meet the needs of different groups and by developing ways to boost the demand for information and its use at various levels of the health care system. This can also be done by developing and testing data collection tools for use at the district level, and provide guidance on the most cost-effective strategies for generating sound data on inequities in health status and health-care coverage.

The achievement of the MDGs (described in Chapter 1) is heavily dependent on robust health systems to deliver health interventions to deal with tuberculosis, malaria, HIV/AIDS, child survival and maternal health. This raises additional issues in relation to health information:

- The need to develop a set of practical "core metrics" to monitor the status and capacity of health systems at the national and sub-national or district level, with special attention given to equity issues. One approach is through Service Availability Mapping (SAM), which is based on a rapid assessment

Table 2.5 Research priorities in health systems financing

Health system financing area	*Research needs and knowledge gaps*	*Comment*
Inputs to health systems	Strengthening national health accounts	More funds are needed for the institutionalization of routine evidence-bases and sound data collection.
	Development and testing of methods to track expenditure by use (e.g. by priority disease, population group, human resources etc.)	Need for improving research on and analysis of all disease-specific health expenditures, expenditures on human resources.
	Financing resources allocation	Need for improving decision-making on balanced health expenditures.
Financing function—revenue collection and pooling	Financing schemes and equity	Which financing scheme to implement for a sound and equitable universal coverage?
	The sustainability of health financing	How to sustain the financing of interventions without relying on donor funding? The search for financing self-sufficiency.
	Health insurance schemes—financing aspects	How to move to universal coverage? What is the role of community insurance in this process?
	Health insurance schemes—administrative and technical aspects	How to manage the administrative costs and the pooling of risks?
	Co-payments, user fees and exemptions	Community participation in the payment of health services: the cost of health services must remain affordable to ensure access to care, while it should prevent unnecessary use of services.
	Public and private mix	What is the role of private insurance schemes? Do they promote more equity?
Financing function—purchasing	The costs, effectiveness and impact on equity of undertaking interventions together, as in real life	Most research focuses on the costs and effects of interventions undertaken by themselves, rather than taking into account interactions. This does not help policy formulation. The impact on health inequalities of interventions also needs to be addressed.
	Human resources, incentives and the rationalization of health services	Health providers must be responsive and accountable to patients. Decisions on the most appropriate incentives to ensure this must be found.
Measurement of key health system outcomes	Routine monitoring and assessment of the impact of the health financing system on access to services. Information on which households face financial catastrophe and impoverishment because of health payment.	This information is critical to develop policies for risk protection.

Source: Evans DB, Health System Financing, Expenditure & Resource Allocation, World Health Organization, 2004.

tool administered through district health management teams that generates a visual representation of disparities in service provision between and within districts. Such a mapping exercise enables district and national planners to use data for public health decision-making.

- The need to develop indicators to monitor the progress to achievement of the MDGs themselves. A baseline of 1990 has been set to attain the MDGs by 2015. The health-related MDGs consist of a few health status indicators and a selected number of health programme coverage indicators. The primary focus on monitoring the MDGs has been on whether a country's indicator trends are on track or not. Research and development efforts are needed to promote better measurement of health-related MDGs and related indicators, especially in low- and middle-income countries with a high burden of disease and poor data.

The Health Metrics Network (HMN) is a newly established global alliance dedicated to meeting the challenges described above. HMN aims to increase the availability and use of timely and accurate health information at sub-national, national and global levels by acting as a catalyst for joint funding and development of core country health information systems. Linking of network activities with the health research system at the country level is essential.

Developing adequate health information systems also means training health-care workers to collect such information. Routine health information in poor countries tends to be collected by large numbers of poorly trained workers, who frequently do not recognize the significance of data collection, or else, collect erroneous data. Research into improving data accuracy in this context would help ensure that data that has been processed would actually help in the assessment of a country's health needs. The efforts of the NGO INDEPTH to mine demographic information through a network of surveillance sites across Africa has yielded disproportionate dividends in understanding patterns of mortality and inequity in health (see Box 2.3).

Regional perspective 2

There is a major need for reliable and timely information on basic indicators pertaining to health systems. This requirement for health systems "benchmarks" was deemed crucial to monitoring and evaluating the achievement of the MDGs, and the performance of the system itself. Included in this is the need for research to develop benchmark indicators for human rights, ethics and equity.

Health services delivery

Little is known about how to scale up health services rapidly in the face of urgent public-health problems and to integrate "vertical", single-disease programmes into the broader health system. There is also a need to do more research on organization and delivery of health services. One priority area relates to developing effective and efficient approaches to dealing with populations that have special needs, such as dispersed rural populations and populations living in urban slums, particularly in order to improve their access to effective services.

More research needs to be done to find ways of helping health workers make sure patients are taking medicines. This knowledge is vital as anti-AIDS programmes are expanded to get antiretrovirals to millions of people who need them in developing countries. There is a need for more research on approaches to improving drug supplies, including cost-recovery schemes and interventions to improve prescribing and dispensing. These interventions should not be restricted to the formal health sector but also include drug retailers who are important providers of health-related products in many countries.

Another priority area is evaluating the development and implementation of strategies to ensure quality in the health system setting. In high-income countries a variety of methods have been used to improve the practice of health

Box 2.3 INDEPTH

To improve the health of the poor it is essential to have adequate information about their health status. Providing such information is the primary focus of the International Network of field sites with continuous Demographic Evaluation of Populations and their Health in developing countries, known as INDEPTH. Aimed at reducing the health inequities worldwide, this network works to maximize global community-based surveillance initiatives in resource-poor countries in the hope that this information might provide a better understanding of the health and social issues faced by these countries.

INDEPTH facilitates cross-site longitudinal health and social studies, introduces methodological and technical workshops, and builds institutional research capacity globally. To gather data on a given population, INDEPTH conducts comparative studies and exchanges experiences on important universal problems. It also creates and shares regional health status assessments and evaluates health interventions in diverse socio-cultural and geographic environments. INDEPTH is also actively involved in recruiting and creating additional sites.

Surveillance data used by INDEPTH, known as the Demographic Surveillance System, offers a mechanism to help countries understand how the health of populations varies from one stage of the health transition in developing countries to another. Such data is also used to evaluate how health equity evolves over time in these countries.

The Demographic Surveillance System is a set of field and computing operations handling the follow-up of primary subjects, such as individuals, households and residential units, and all their related health and demographic factors within a specific geographic region. This system also defines risk and corresponding trends in birth, death, and migration rates in a population over a certain period of time. The system's ability to track individuals over time has made it possible to conduct population-based controlled experiments on the impact that new drugs, vaccines and changes in health service delivery systems have had on morbidity and mortality. Such demographic surveillance has been invaluable in providing information on the correlation between social and economic status and health outcomes.

With 36 demographic surveillance system field sites in 19 countries in Africa, Asia, Oceania, and Central America, INDEPTH is essentially a scientific and policy forum for the development and assessment of health equity strategies catering to the needs of the developing world.

For more information visit: www.indepth-network.org

professionals, including clinical guidelines, continuing education, the use of computers in assisting diagnosis, and audit and feedback by professional societies. However, a very small proportion of such studies has been undertaken in low-income countries.

The rise of HIV/AIDS, tuberculosis, and malaria in tandem with noncommunicable diseases in many parts of the world has highlighted the need for better systems to manage chronic disease. This will require health systems to develop capacities to facilitate continuity of care, support self-management, and provide decision support for health workers that is consistent with scientific evidence and patient preferences. It should also ensure information systems that will provide, for example, timely reminders to health personnel and patients, and feedback on performance to health-care providers. Cost effective approaches to developing and implementing chronic disease management systems in low-income countries are urgently needed.

Regional perspective 3

A major priority for health systems research should be research into the development of policies for scaling up health services to meet contemporary health challenges (e.g. achieving the MDGs). It should include research on how to better integrate "vertical", single-disease programmes within the broader health system.

Regional perspective 4

Further research is needed on regulatory aspects, corruption and poor governance within health systems in resource-poor countries.

2.4 Future challenges

New tools and methodologies needed

Few people appreciate how important it is to develop new tools and methodologies to tackle a given research problem or realize that new research can bridge gaps in current research. Systematic reviews, which are usually used to evaluate the effectiveness of health interventions, should also be used to evaluate the findings of research on health policy and health systems. Some work in this area to improve clinical practice, for example, should be acknowledged and built upon *(16, 17)*. Shifting contexts of the environment in which health systems operate also necessitates a review of currently available research tools.

The previous sections have highlighted that information and core metrics to monitor the status and capacity of health systems at national and sub-national levels are critical for health systems research. Some work has already been done in this area *(18)* and various tools and methodologies have been developed. This includes, among others, CHOICE (CHOosing Interventions that are Cost-Effective), Marginal Budgeting for Bottlenecks (MBB), and tools for analysing the health workforce. However, considering the changing context and landscape of major global health problems, there is perhaps a need to revisit these tools and consider developing more practical, feasible and sustainable measures and benchmarks for health system functions that include building of national capacities to collect the necessary information.

Also, current methodologies in health systems research are often criticized for being less than rigorous and as sub-standard science. A gold standard methodological equivalent of the randomized controlled trial in clinical research, or the positive-negative control design of experimental biomedical research, continues to elude this field.

Part of the problem is that methodologies which were developed for other fields of research have been adopted in health systems research, even though they may be unsuitable or inappropriate. The answer does not lie in adapting or adopting these to the field of health systems research but rather in investing in innovative ways to study health systems. Some advances are already being made to create such new approaches.

While acknowledging that causal chains in public health interventions are complex, some have suggested that a "plausibility" approach may provide valid evidence of the impact of programmes or interventions *(19)*. This would mean developing causal statements using observational designs with a comparison group. Methodologies are also becoming available to examine socioeconomic disparities in health conditions and service delivery *(20)*. Such an approach, called "programme-incidence" or "coverage-inequality" analysis, facilitates studies that aim to assess how well health programmes are reaching the poor. The latter approach is used to determine distribution of programme outputs across socioeconomic groups within the target population, instead of standard cost-benefit analysis where outputs are analysed relative to unit of input *(21)*. Another example from Canada illustrates an innovative, multi-disciplinary effort to develop a conceptual framework to study social organization and its impact on health status (see Box 2.4).

Raising the profile and sending a signal

There is an inherent tension in health systems research between the need for more fundamental work to develop better tools and more robust conceptual frameworks and the preferred focus on more local, context-specific, applied and community-based participatory research. Clearly, both fundamental and local research are needed and should complement each other. And although the context-specific, local approach may seem more relevant, attention should also be given to fundamental research as it may disproportionately raise the profile of the field as a whole, thus sending a strong signal to the scientific community of a willingness to explore new vistas and novel ideas.

For this to happen, the development of new conceptual frameworks, tools and methodologies that reach beyond traditional scientific disciplines is needed. Health systems research must be ready to learn from the frontier areas of science in general, such as systems science, chaos theory, social organization research, bioinformatics, the use of "scenarios" and neural networks. For example, a major development in the post-genomics era is the emergence of systems biology as a key scientific discipline to understand complex interac-

Box 2.4 Studying how societies optimize human health and well-being

Inspired by the question: "Why are there persistent differences in the health of children within countries and between nations which cannot be attributed to the quality of health care or living standards?", a project known as Successful Societies was launched in 2002 by the Canadian Institute for Advanced Research (CIAR).

This innovative research project explores the social processes underlying key health and human development outcomes within populations and, on a broader level, the social conditions that underpin the collective development of social communities on a national and local level.

Collective development refers to the capacity of society, at any level, to develop features fundamentally tied to social well-being, including social equality, access to political participation, cultural tolerance, social inclusion, and access to education and employment.

The programme will attempt to seek answers to some key questions, including:

- What kind of social conditions matter?
- How do the social relations in a community affect the capacities and well-being of the individuals who are part of it?
- What types of social relations are most conducive to effective development, both of the community and of the people who live in it?

Drawing on experiences of diverse events such as the course of the AIDS epidemic in Africa, rates of crime in Chicago, and the fate of the Roma (gypsies) in Europe, the strategies to be used will include mobilizing existing research, promoting interaction among scholars in various fields, and conducting new comparative empirical research to assess the impact of key features of social relations in local, national, and regional contexts.

Successful Societies brings together individuals working in cultural studies, epidemiology, developmental psychology, cultural and political sociology, philosophy, history, and areas on the boundary between economics and political science. The idea is to take an interdisciplinary exchange approach to advance the research frontier in theoretical and empirical terms.

For more information visit: www.ciar.ca

Source: Canadian Institute for Advanced Research, Annual Report, 2002–2003.

tion in biological systems. This field aims to "sift through a deluge of data in search of coherent patterns of stimulus and response" *(22)*. The parallel with a health system is not far-fetched. The involvement of these disciplines would not only improve the standing of health systems research as a whole but also the quality of its science. At the same time as exploring these frontiers, however, health systems research must keep its feet firmly on the ground and interact more effectively with the broader health research system. This is the subject of Chapter 3.

Vannevar Bush's *Endless Frontier (23)* (see Section 1.2) laid the foundations for the boom in basic scientific research in post-Second World War America. Now is the time to lay the foundations for a new era of research into health systems.

Building capacity

All the above must be complemented by a strong effort to build capacity and effective institutions for health systems research to flourish. Capacity building efforts should pay close attention to the role of mentors and teachers in nurturing the next generation of health systems researchers. Within institutions, an environment should be created that would attract the best people by providing attractive academic career structures, incentives (financial and otherwise), access to information, and opportunities to teach, do research, and participate in meetings and courses.

A call for action

Health systems research is in need of a new paradigm. The future cannot be business as usual. For health systems research to be elevated to the same status as molecular biology and genomics, substantial and sustainable resources and support must be mobilized. A "grand challenges" approach should be considered for health systems research, as has been done with biomedical research, to develop interventions to deal with global health challenges *(24)*.

However, it is not just about more funding. It requires a concomitant commitment and passion from the health systems research community itself, and a willingness to think creatively and be more open to new ideas. Unless this happens, health systems research may be unable to escape the den of scientific poverty and inequity.

References

1. *The World Health Report 2003—Shaping the Future*. Geneva, World Health Organization, 2003.
2. Joint Learning Initiative in Human Resources for Health and Development *Working for Health: a Strategy Report*. New York, NY, in press.
3. Stilwell B et al. Migration of health-care workers from developing countries: strategic approaches to its management. *Bulletin of the World Health Organization*, 2004, 82:595–600.
4. Pang T et al. Brain drain and health professionals. *British Medical Journal*, 2002, 324:499–500.
5. Woods N. Global health governance: reconciling macroeconomic stability with a major

scaling-up of aid to combat HIV/AIDS in low-income countries. Oxford, Global Economic Governance Programme, Report of meeting held on June 22, 2004.
6. Xu K et al. Household catastrophic health expenditure: a multicountry analysis. *Lancet*, 2003, 362:111–117.
7. Evans T, Stansfield S. Health information in the new millennium: a gathering storm. *Bulletin of the World Health Organization*, 2003, 81:856.
8. Travis P et al. Overcoming health systems constraints to achieve the millennium development goals. *Lancet*, 2004, 364:900–906.
9. *Strengthening Health Systems: The role and promise of policy and systems research*, Geneva, Alliance for Health Policy and Systems Research, 2004.
10. Nuyens Y. Health systems research and the World Health Organization. Document prepared for WHO/EIP, Geneva, April 2004.
11. Andreano R. *The International Health Policy Programme: An Internal Assessment*. Madison, WI, University of Wisconsin Press, 2001.
12. Janovsky K (ed). Health policy and systems development: an agenda for research. Geneva, World Health Organization, 1996.
13. *The 10/90 Report on Health Research, 2003–2004*. Geneva, Global Forum for Health Research, 2004.
14. Shine K. National strategies for organizing health services research. Presentation at International Conference on the Scientific Basis of Health Services, Washington, DC, September 20–23, 2003.
15. Task Force on Health Systems Research. Informed choices for attaining the millennium development goals: towards an international cooperative agenda for health systems research. *Lancet*, 2004, 364:997–1003.
16. Oxman A et al. No magic bullets: a systematic review of 102 trials of hypertension to improve professional practice. *Canadian Medical Association Journal,* 1995, 153:1423–1431.
17. Grimshaw J et al. Changing provider behaviour: an overview of systematic reviews of interventions. Medical Care, 2001, 39 (suppl. 2): 112–45.
18. *The World Health Report 2000—Health Systems: Improving Performance*. Geneva, World Health Organization, 2000.
19. Victora C et al. Evidence-based public health: moving beyond randomized trials. *American Journal of Public Health*, 2004, 94:400–405.
20. Schellenberg JA et al. Inequities among the very poor: health care for children in rural Southern Tanzania. *Lancet*, 2003, 361:561–566.
21. Gwatkin D. How well do health programmes reach the poor? *Lancet*, 2003, 361:540–541.
22. Pennisi E. Systems biology-tracing life's circuitry. *Science*, 2003, 302:1646–1649.
23. Bush V. *Science: The Endless Frontier*. A report to the President by Vannevar Bush, Director of the Office of Scientific Research and Development. Washington, DC, US Government Printing Office, 1945.
24. Varmus H. Grand challenges in global health. *Science*, 2003, 302:398–399.

3

Strengthening Health Research Systems

"Research is a system involving people, institutions and processes. Its pursuit depends on systematic analysis, creativity and exploration."
(Commission on Health Research for Development)

"The health research system is the brains of the health system: it is a tool to organize, understand, operate and improve it."
(Prawase Wasi)

Key Messages

- Leadership, funding, researchers and institutions, and the capacity to utilize research findings are as important as new discoveries.
- National health research should focus on priority health problems in the country concerned, on health system challenges and on managing opportunities for future growth and development. International efforts should support strategic research opportunities in particular.
- Research agendas should be set up to succeed. This means adequate, sustainable and transparent funding, professional research managers, ethical standards, and accountability in the use of public funds.
- In addition to peer reviewed journal articles in large, international databases, other forms of research have potential value and should be recognized.
- Funds should also be invested in strengthening human and institutional research capacities to address complex health problems.
- Biomedical discoveries cannot improve

Interesting numbers

10%	Percentage of research outputs produced by health researchers surveyed in 13 low- and middle-income countries that were referenced in international databases of journal articles.
22,000	Estimated number of scientific journals in the world in 2002.
1/3	Proportion of researchers, policy-makers and other users of research in 13 low- and middle-income countries who said in a survey that there was either no rational process to set health research priorities in their countries, or that they were unaware of how priorities were identified or set.
20,000	Number of qualified professionals emigrating annually from Africa since 1990.
3%	Percentage of public sector funding from developing countries directed towards health research, as a proportion of total global spending on health research.

(Sources for these numbers are given on the report web site: www.who.int/rpc/wr2004)

people's health without research to find out how to apply these within different health systems, population groups, and diverse political and social contexts.

- The culture and practice of health research should be expanded beyond academic institutions and laboratories to include health service providers, policy-makers and civil society.

3.1 What is commonly known about health research activities?

What some people can count easily

People interested in scientific performance often look at the number of scientific articles published in peer reviewed journals. This is easily done. Basic information and summaries of many articles are available in large reference databases covering scientific research from many countries on a wide range of topics. In 2000 alone, for example, the Thomson Institute for Scientific Information's (ISI) databases included over 365,000 articles that were published in more than 3,200 scientific journals addressing a broad range of health topics—not only biomedical research—written by scientists and health researchers working in 175 countries.

There are reasons for wanting to count the number of scientific publications. Firstly, such numbers can be linked to the research capacity and knowledge pool of an individual, institution, country, region or even the world as a whole. For example, using the ISI database, Figure 3.1 illustrates the proportion of scientific publications on health topics written by authors in seven regions of the world. This shows that Europe, the Western Pacific and the United States account for approximately 90% of scientific output on health *(1)*.

Secondly, the number of scientific articles published in peer reviewed journals is an alluring figure because some argue that at the national level, the number of scientific articles, especially those addressing biomedical research topics, reflect financial investments in research and development within a country. But given the difficulties of estimating government, business, and foreign investments in health research and development, particularly in low- and middle-income countries, counting published articles alone is not a sufficient approach to estimate health research expenditure.

Is counting articles enough to shape health research policy and investment?

No. Although newspaper articles and scientific production in peer reviewed journals may provide some indication of research capacity or of the knowledge pool, the research process is far more complex. It spans the entire spectrum of policies related to knowledge creation as well as its diffusion and use. It cannot be captured by one figure or by quantitative measures alone. Particularly for low- and middle-income countries, focusing narrowly on the number of

Figure 3.1 Proportion of scientific publications addressing health topics from different regions* in the world, 2001

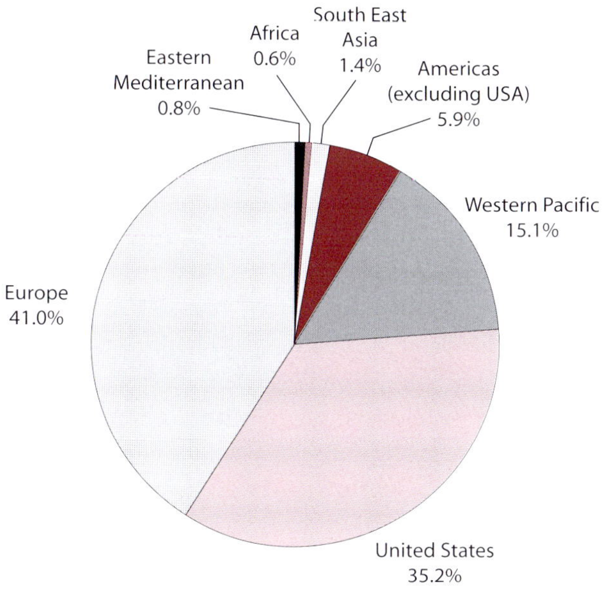

Source: World Health Organization, 2004, based on Institute for Scientific Information (ISI)'s Science Citation Index (SCI) database from 2001.

* WHO regional structure, about 15% of these articles have authors working in more than one country, and in this case, each country gets part of the "credit" for the article.

peer reviewed research articles—or on some variation such as the proportion of highly-cited articles—has many pitfalls. There is much debate on whether reference databases are representative of all research articles that have been published globally. Another issue is whether journals tend to publish research on health topics primarily concerning high-income countries. Finally, there are questions as to whether the peer review process itself stifles innovation and is not necessarily a guarantor of quality.

In fact, peer reviewed journal articles referenced in large, international databases are only one type of research output. In an interview-based survey of almost 1,900 individuals identified as active health researchers in 13 low- and middle-income countries, a much wider range of research outputs were reported for the period 1998–2002 *(2)*. Pooling data collected across countries, the expanded list includes peer reviewed journal articles referenced in international databases (about 10% of total research productivity); peer reviewed journal articles referenced in regional or national databases (about 20%); conference presentations (about 26%); books, non-peer reviewed articles and unpublished manuscripts (about 24%); as well as outputs that are not just for other researchers, such as policy reports, press releases and other media items (about 20%). Also, more than 10% of these researchers reported having registered a national or international patent. The majority of those with registered patents worked in clinical or biomedical research.

In addition to the various forms of "explicit" knowledge mentioned above, it is important to note that knowledge can/is also generated by a variety of players not strictly within formal research processes or as presented in publications. It is likely that a wealth of "tacit" knowledge already exists to be drawn upon during the research process. Also, much of the results of research are probably applied in practice without first having to publish them in the traditional manner. Timeliness, responsiveness to needs of users and a focus on coming up with strategic solutions are as important as precision, rigour and detailed analysis.

THERE IS BASIC, THERE IS APPLIED AND THERE IS STRATEGIC RESEARCH

Most people know about basic and applied research. In truth, research spans a spectrum starting from basic, fundamental research to applied research and extends to operational and management research. In this report's context, the question is: what type(s) of research are relevant and important in bridging the gap between what is known and what is actually being done?

Research has struggled with the goals of "knowing" and understanding ("basic" research) on the one hand, and with "doing" and using ("applied" research) on the other. There is also a perception that the former is more likely to be "universal" or "global" in nature and performed in the developed world, and the latter more "local" and focused on national priorities. In his landmark treatise *(3)*, Stokes concluded that the traditional distinction between basic and applied research is inadequate and too limiting, and that a category called "strategic" research ("Pasteur's quadrant") needs to be added. This is research leading to "results of evident interest to a broad class of users, external to the research community, that can be identified at the time the research is funded; intended users of the research may also be within the research community". Strategic research is also characterized by the fact that it draws on global knowledge for solving local problems (see Figure 3.2). It is also important to emphasize the rationale for having the local-applied quadrant, e.g. that a genomics institute is not needed in every country. The role of strategic research is revisited in Section 3.3. below.

The focus of strategic research on users may make it most relevant for translating knowledge into actions to improve health. The success of strategic research depends, to some extent, on maximizing the impact of explicit and tacit knowledge within health systems and can gain much from a "knowledge management" framework in public health. This is defined as a set of principles and tools to optimize and integrate the iterative processes of creating, developing, disseminating and applying knowledge for strategic problem-solving and organizational effectiveness in the field of public health. The scaling up of knowledge management efforts in public health will be important for translating research and evidence into policy, practice and social transformation.

WHAT IS NEEDED TO PROVIDE A MORE COMPLETE PICTURE?

To understand whether research produces knowledge that improves health, it

Figure 3.2 A view of strategic research

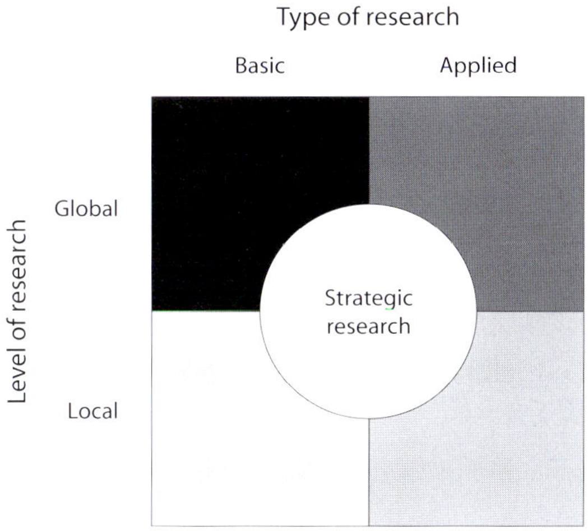

Darkness of quadrants indicate approximate, relative intensities of activity and levels of funding support. Global-basic quadrant funded primarily by developed countries; global-applied quadrant by industry; local-basic and local-applied by public and external donor agencies in developing countries. Strategic research straddles all four quadrants and combines global and local activities.

Source: A. Pablos-Mendez, Knowledge Management and Sharing, World Health Organization, Geneva.

is not enough to simply look at the number of papers produced. Other issues need to be considered, such as:

- How are research topics selected and by whom?
- How are research activities financed?
- Who are the people and institutions involved in producing and synthesizing research?
- What are the different values and objectives of those involved in health research?
- To what extent are potential beneficiaries involved in the research process?
- How are research results disseminated and to whom?
- How is research used to make products, interventions and generate information for better health?
- How are research activities evaluated and made accountable to society?

Most countries need to adopt a more comprehensive and participatory approach to health research in order to develop policies and strategies to better ensure that research produced attains its goal of improving health outcomes. This is the underlying premise of a "health research system".

3.2 What is a system for health research and why is it important?

The system for health research, which was introduced in Chapter 1, refers to the people, institutions and activities involved in the generation and application of knowledge to promote, restore and/or maintain the health status of populations. It also includes the mechanisms that can be adopted to encourage the utilization of health research. While health research systems can operate at local, national, regional or global levels, this chapter focuses on national health research systems to highlight the importance of countries producing their own research and using existing research to identify and address their health problems.

The four main functions of a health research system are essential to attain the goals of knowledge for better health:

1. stewardship—strong leadership to direct, coordinate, manage and review health research;
2. financing—sustainable and transparent processes to mobilize and allocate funds for research;
3. resources—sufficient human and institutional capacities to produce and especially to use research;
4. producing and using research—producing research that addresses health challenges, synthesizing research results, and using the knowledge gained, particularly within health systems.

WHY IS A SYSTEMS APPROACH TO HEALTH RESEARCH IMPORTANT?

On a national scale, health research efforts are often hindered by insufficient coordination. Research activities in various health-related fields can be fragmented, isolated from each other and wastefully competitive. Moreover, there is often little communication and consultation between the producers of research and the users of research: policy-makers, health providers, civil society, the private sector, other researchers, and the general public.

A well-coordinated, systematic approach to health research involves all stakeholders. For instance, efforts to increase the quality, relevance and production of research also need to consider whether there is a demand for this research.

Countries need a health research system to identify priorities, mobilize resources and maximize the use of existing ones, develop and sustain the human and institutional capacity necessary to conduct research, disseminate research results to target audiences, apply research results in policy and practice, and evaluate the impact of research on health outcomes. More systematized approaches to these processes involved in the performance and production of health research would help to improve the transparency and accountability of health research activities.

The health research system and the health system cannot exist in separate worlds. The notion of "knowledge for better health" demands that the health research system should provide more direction to strengthen the health system. Health research can provide guidance on how to invest limited resources allocated to health systems more effectively. Health research must also investigate a broad range of issues in addition to life sciences or clinical medicine, such as:

- what makes us healthy or ill, including a broad range of social, environmental and economic determinants;
- how to prevent illness, accidents, injuries, and how to treat these more effectively and efficiently;
- how to be responsive to people's needs and expectations;
- how to provide services for all kinds of peoples, groups and sub-populations, particularly those who have been chronically underserved or simply not covered at all;
- how to take into account that individuals live and experience health and illness within households, communities and social networks;
- how to organize health services given the existence of different administrative, geographic and political levels;
- how to obtain accurate and reliable basic health information;
- how to set health priorities and goals and develop strategies to implement them;
- how to train an appropriate mix of health professionals and health workers;
- how to finance the health system in an equitable and sustainable manner;
- how to mix preventive and curative services, private and public services, disease specific services and more comprehensive services;
- how to link the health research system with the non-health public and private sectors;
- how to involve people and institutions in the process;
- how to evaluate health systems.

These questions may not be exhaustive, but they are relevant to all countries and all health systems. All countries, especially those with relatively limited resources, need evidence and knowledge to shape health policy. Research on health systems, the topic of Chapter 2, should be viewed as an investment and not a cost.

Does a system's perspective need further development?

Yes. The main conclusions of a recent review based on more than 45 case studies written since 2000—from some 35 low- and middle-income countries—underscored the need to regard health research as a functional system *(4)* with elements working towards a common goal. For example, poor coordination between research institutions at national, regional and international levels is the main obstacle to effective functioning of the health research system.

Studies show that many countries have no national health research agenda or mechanism to coordinate these activities. They show that stakeholders do not participate in the development or implementation of research policies. The studies also found that overall demand for research was low and that there was a lack of accessibility to research findings.

These case studies suggest the need for a systems approach to the organization of health research, irrespective of the national context. Yet these studies do not always provide enough guidance on which policy options would be more appropriate to strengthen national health research systems. Moreover, qualitative case studies may not cover all aspects of a health research system and make it difficult to see changes over time or across different national settings.

Many excellent reports and studies on health research activities include quantitative data (see Box 3.1). Most focus selectively on specific scientific fields, institutions or actors. This is partly because data that covers all health research activities—which is more than medical research and yet less than all scientific research and development—is often not readily available even in most high-income countries.

A summary of the functions and operational components of a health research system is presented in Table 3.1. Further details of each function—stewardship, finances, resources, and producing and using research—as well as approaches on how to understand and potentially strengthen each are explored in the following four sections of this chapter.

Box 3.1 Evaluating biomedical research in the United States

In the United States, the National Academy of Sciences, the umbrella organization for the National Academy of Engineering, the Institute of Medicine and the National Research Council, released a report in 2003 entitled: *Large-Scale Biomedical Science*.

The report presented recommendations on how to improve the US government's approach to large-scale biomedical research, on how best to advance knowledge and on how to produce innovations that would benefit society. The report presented the following recommendations:

1. Assessing research proposals: The National Institutes of Health (NIH) have no formal mechanism for assessing opportunities for biomedical research by comparing, evaluating and ranking research programmes. Criteria to evaluate competing scientific initiatives were, however, proposed in 1988. These were divided into three categories: scientific merit, social benefits and programmatic concerns.

   The report takes these proposals a step further by recommending the implementation of an open and systematic method across the NIH for soliciting and reviewing biomedical research proposals. It said that this should be part of the priority-setting process to determine the allocation of federal funds.
2. Evaluating research outcomes: The White House Office of Management and Budget is trying to impose stricter performance criteria for federal research agencies which hope to receive funding for research projects. The *Large-Scale Biomedical Science* report explores the debate about whether or not basic research can be evaluated. Critics of the evaluation of basic research argue that outcomes cannot be measured on a regular basis because they are unpredictable. Moreover, there is often a time lag between the generation of knowledge and its application in practice. On the other hand, proponents of the evaluation of biomedical research findings argue that at least some benchmarking of quality, relevance and leadership is needed to provide some indication of the potential usefulness of a research programme. The report also recommends that federal funding agencies should conduct a thorough analysis of their recent large-scale biomedical research initiatives once they are well established, to evaluate their effectiveness and efficiency in achieving their goals.

Source: *Large-scale biomedical science: exploring strategies for future research*. The Institute of Medicine and the National Research Council of the National Academies. Washington DC: The National Academies Press, 2003.

3.3 Stewardship: what can good leadership do?

Effective management and coordination are crucial for health research to address a country's health problems as well as other health challenges found around the world. Sound governance in health research is needed at the national level to connect health challenges, research priorities and practical approaches to improve health. Throughout the world, there are different systems for managing and coordinating research. For instance, in the Islamic Republic of Iran, the Department of Research and Technology at the Ministry of Health and Medical Education is the body that implements health research policies through the Medical Commission of the National Research Council. In Pakistan, it is the Pakistan Medical Research Council (PMRC) that performs stewardship functions on behalf of the Ministry of Health, which has administrative control of the PMRC.

No one organizational structure is appropriate for health research in all countries. But it is important for all countries to understand the current structures, strengths and potential challenges facing leadership in health research, as well as the range of stakeholders involved in the national health research process. An example of this is the many key stakeholders within the Malaysian health research system listed in Figure 3.3. The Philippines has also recently reviewed the way in which health research is organized in the country (see Box 3.2).

The following areas of leadership and management are essential regardless of the organizational structure of the health research system:

- Creating a vision for integrating national health research with the health system.

Table 3.1 Summary of the functions and operational components of health research systems

Functions	*Operational components*
Stewardship	■ Define and articulate vision for national health research system (HRS) ■ Identify appropriate health research priorities and coordinate adherence to them ■ Set and monitor ethical standards for health research and research partnerships ■ Monitor and evaluate the HRS
Financing	Secure research funds and allocate them accountably
Creating and sustaining resources	Build, strengthen, and sustain the human and physical capacity to conduct, absorb, and utilize health research
Producing and using research	■ Produce scientifically valid outputs ■ Translate and communicate research to inform health policy, strategies, practices, and public opinion ■ Promote the use of research to develop new tools (drugs, vaccines, devices, and other applications) to improve health

Source: Pang T et al. Knowledge for better health—a conceptual framework and foundation for health research systems. *Bulletin of the World Health Organization*, 2003, 81:815–820.

- Setting and adhering to appropriate health research priorities.
- Emphasizing strategic research and management of knowledge.
- Setting and monitoring ethical standards for health research and research partnerships.
- Monitoring and evaluating all the elements of the system to improve it.

Good leadership is required to coordinate and implement national priorities for health research. Given that resources for research are limited, particularly in low-income countries, it is important that they are directed towards research activities that would optimize health benefits, hence the notion of "knowledge for better health". This means identifying health problems of greatest national interest where increased funds, capacities, and innovative approaches would attain better health in an equitable fashion. For example, Australia, Canada, New Zealand (see Box 3.3) and the United States have set specific health

Figure 3.3 Key stakeholders within Malaysia's national health research system

Funders	Producers	Evaluators/Monitors	Users
National	Government Research Institutions	Ministry of Health	Ministry of Health
Ministry of Health	Public Universities	Ministry of Science, Technology & Environment	Health Service Providers (public and private)
Other Ministries	Private Universities	Universities	Ministries
International	Ministry of Health Departments	International Agencies	Universities
Pharmaceutical Companies	Industries	National Committee on Clinical Research	International
Industries	Corporatized Government Research Institutions	Government Research Institutions	Pharmaceutical Companies
Professional Organizations	Professional Organizations	Corporatized Government Research Institutions	Researchers
NGOs	NGOs	Foreign Research Institutions	NGOs
General Public	Foreign Research Institutions	Private Medical Institutions	Professional Organizations
	Private Medical Institutions	Ethics Committees	General Public
			Media
			Industries

Source: Institute for Health Systems Research, Ministry of Health, Kuala Lumpur, Malaysia.

research priorities and strategies for indigenous populations who tend to suffer from worse health outcomes than the non-indigenous populations.

Various systematic approaches and tools have been created to coordinate health research priorities at national levels. One example of a mechanism for priority setting or coordination is the Essential National Health Research (ENHR) strategy. This strategy is based on consensus-building among a broad range of stakeholders, including: researchers, policy-makers, health-care providers and community representatives.

Another method is a matrix approach that combines economic and institutional perspectives in a single tool. This was developed by the Global Forum for Health Research, the NGO that has brought the 10/90 gap in health research to the fore. The matrix approach looks at disease burden, determinants for the persistence of that burden, present level of knowledge, cost-effectiveness, and resource flows. These are discussed in relation to individuals, families and

Box 3.2 Creating a national health research system in the Philippines

The Philippines started to reorganize its health research system recently by creating a new body called the Philippine National Health Research System. Created by the Department of Health (DOH) and the Department of Science and Technology (DOST), the new body seeks to encourage other stakeholders such as universities, civil society groups and NGOs, business and foundations, and expatriate communities to play a greater role in health research.

Revised Structure of Health Research in the Philippines

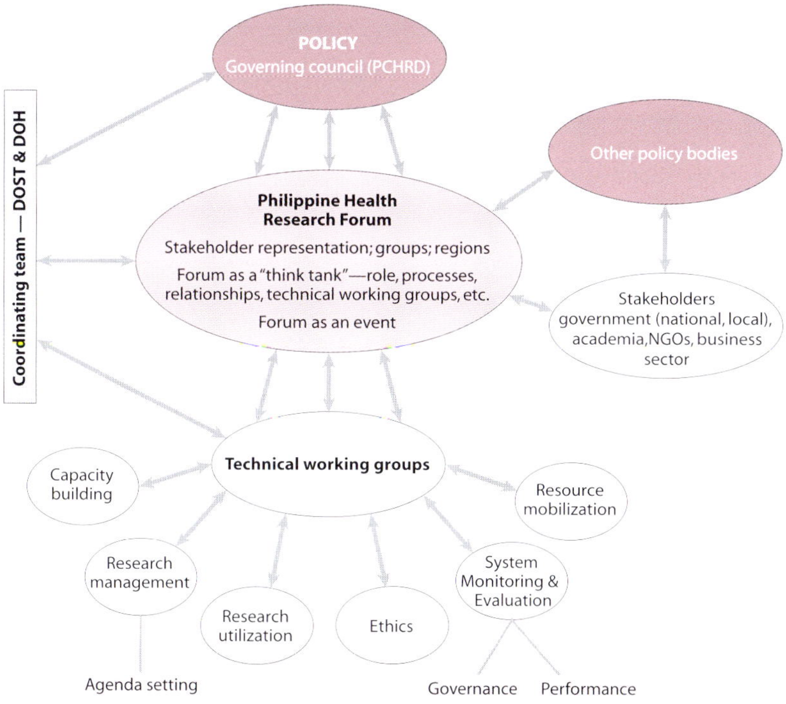

This body replaced the Philippine Council for Health Research and Development (PCHRD) which was created in 1982 as the policy-making body of the national health research system. The PCHRD was the first major organization established in the Philippines to coordinate and lead national health research.

To create the country's new national health research system, a working group was set up to provide the framework for its structure, organization, and monitoring and evaluation. The working group recommended two options for reorganizing the national health research system. In the first model, its structure would be akin to a virtual organization, respecting the formal authority of the existing agencies that comprise the health research system. In the second model, called "nodal governance," the national health research system would identify natural nodes of research networks, interlink them, and lead them towards certain objectives. Both models built on existing health research structures to reduce bureaucratic hurdles entailed in the restructuring.

The working group finally proposed that all regions adopt the structure outlined to the left to reorganize the national health research system, to ensure that all sectors in this model are represented.

Source: Proceedings & Highlights of Philippine National Health Research System (draft), Philippine National Health Research System Monograph Series, Technical Working Group on System Structure, Organization, Monitoring and Evaluation, 2004.

Box 3.3 New Zealand: health research for Maori by Maori

One in seven people in New Zealand identify themselves as being of Maori origin. The Health Research Council of New Zealand (HRC) recognizes that, as a governmental body, it has a role in ensuring that Maori, as *tangata whenua* or the indigenous people of New Zealand, have access to and are able to utilize the resources available to improve their health status. The founding document of New Zealand, the Treaty of Waitangi, recognizes that Maori tribes and sub-tribes have authority over their involvement in health research. This document also states that Maori should expect the same standard of health as non-Maori, and an equitable share of benefits from government spending on health care.

The HRC launched an initiative called the Health Research Strategy to Improve Maori Health and Well-being 2004–2008 with the goal of improving Maori health by funding high-quality health research based on Maori health priorities and needs. The present strategy builds on a previous initiative, called the Maori Health Research Strategic Plan for 1998–2002. Under the new scheme:

- The HRC identified Maori as a priority population and area for more investment. As a result, all nine HRC research portfolios highlight health needs and relevance to Maori.
- The HRC developed a research portfolio that supports a "by Maori for Maori" *Kaupapa** and aims to build Maori capability to undertake health research, prioritize the development of Maori science, paradigms and methodologies, and ensure *Kaupapa* Maori-focused research is funded.
- Maori health research is also carried out through other health research portfolios.
- All applicants to the HRC for funding need to demonstrate that their research is responsive to the needs and diversity of Maori, which entails consultation with Maori representatives. If research is of interest to Maori, then the design and conduct of the research, the storage of samples or data and the dissemination of research findings will be undertaken in a manner that reflects Maori knowledge and values.
- The HRC Board includes two Maori members.
- The Maori Health Committee participates with the other Research Committees to develop policy and process recommendations to the HRC.
- Joint ventures have been established with other public entities to invest in Maori development research as part of the HRC's Partnership Programme.
- The HRC's investment in Maori health research has increased and now represents more than 9% of its total investment in health research.

Additional areas in the present strategic plan include:

- developing the ability of indigenous people's communities to undertake research projects;
- ensuring that Maori health research is innovative and opportunities to contribute to economic goals are exploited where appropriate;
- ensuring that Maori have the ability to engage in the debate on the development and implementation of new health research technologies;
- ensuring that research collaboration with other indigenous groups are fostered;
- ensuring that Maori ethical issues are part of the discussion on health ethics.

For more information, visit:

www.hrc.govt.nz/assets/pdfs/policy/framework.pdf

www.hrc.govt.nz/assets/pdfs/publications/Strategic%20Plan%202004-2008.pdf

* Kaupapa Maori research uses tools which are based on Maori paradigms and methodologies. This represents an important part of the development of Maori thought, culture and world-view.

Source: The Health Research Council of New Zealand, March 2004. Ngā Pou Rangahau Hauora Kia Whakapiki Ake Te Hauora Māori 2004–2008. The Health Research Strategy to Improve Maori Health and Well-being 2004–2008.

communities as well as ministries of health, research institutions and health systems. These areas are also discussed with regard to health; central government and macro-economic policies; and put in a global context.

A survey of more than 550 policy-makers and almost 1,900 researchers in 13 low- and middle-income countries in 2004 found that, on average, a greater proportion of policy-makers than researchers reported that more resources should be spent on health systems research such as health policy, service delivery, financing and surveillance as the best means of meeting the objectives of the national health research system *(5)*. In contrast, a greater share of researchers said more should be spent on basic research to meet those goals. The amount researchers said was needed was greater than the amount policy-makers said they would allocate.

Moreover, a greater share of policy-makers than of researchers surveyed wanted more funds spent on policy-driven or commissioned research based on identified priorities to meet the objectives of the national health research system in an efficient way. In contrast, researchers wanted to allocate a greater proportion on researcher-driven research, meaning research reflecting the researcher's scientific interests, rather than with what policy-makers would allocate to this type of research to meet the same goals.

More striking is that about a third of policy-makers, researchers and users of research interviewed said that there was either no rational process to set health research priorities in their country or that they were unaware of how priorities were identified or set (see Figure 3.4). This finding supports case study findings mentioned earlier on the absence of mechanisms to coordinate health research. The message is clear: within each country, a better awareness and understanding of different perspectives may inform national dialogue and processes to identify and coordinate health research priorities and their implementation.

Another dimension to consider when coordinating priorities is the immediate focus of research, as this can differ considerably. For example, health research activities can address basic or fundamental questions, develop

Figure 3.4 Perspectives on research priority setting processes

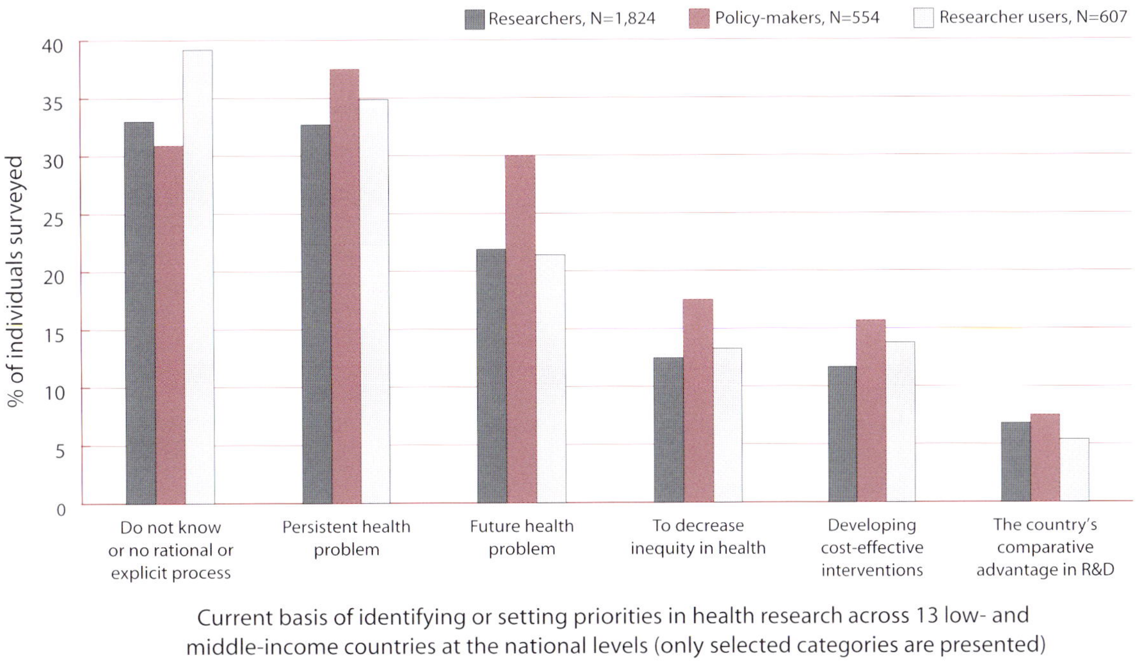

Source: Health Research Systems Analyses Initiative, World Health Organization, 2004.

applications and products, or concentrate on specific managerial and operational challenges. In fact, many ask what is the right mix of basic and applied research activities within a national health research system. Rather than getting bogged down in this traditional debate, good leadership and research management should promote strategic research *(3)* (see Figure 3.2). This means that from the start, not only are the relevant questions and appropriate methods convincing, but the potential health benefits and the people who would benefit are also clearly specified.

Moreover a clear vision and strong social pressure are needed to create incentives for public and private sectors to work more closely together towards mutual objectives (see Box 3.4). In fact, recent success with public-private partnerships looking at neglected diseases is an example of international strategic

Box 3.4 Public-private partnerships for research and development

Public-private partnerships (PPPs) have proved to be an innovative approach to the discovery, development and provision of drugs and vaccines. There are mutual benefits for the public and private sectors in pooling their resources and technologies in research and development (R&D). The public sector stands to gain more business credibility and authority, increased resources and access to private sector skills and management talents *(1)*. The private sector, in turn, may benefit from more corporate influence in national and global policy-making, tax breaks, market penetration, as well as brand and image promotion.

Four notable examples of PPPs are described below. While most of their activities relate to R&D, the ultimate goal of these partnerships is to ensure that these products reach poor patients in developing countries.

The Medicines for Malaria Venture was created in 1999 by WHO and IFPMA (International Federation of Pharmaceuticals Manufacturers Associations). It seeks to bring together public, private and philanthropic partners to fund and manage the discovery, development and registration of affordable and appropriate antimalarial drugs for disease-endemic countries. Its strategy is to build on existing knowledge by combining the expertise of the pharmaceutical industry in drug discovery and development with that of the public sector in biology, clinical medicine, field experience and its public responsibility.

The International AIDS Vaccine Initiative was established in 1996 and works to speed the development and worldwide distribution of AIDS vaccines. Its activities fall in four key categories: 1) a scientific programme, which seeks to accelerate the development of new and innovative AIDS vaccines; 2) education and advocacy programmes, to mobilize international support for an AIDS vaccine; 3) encouraging industrial participation in AIDS vaccine development; and 4) providing global access to AIDS vaccines.

The Global Alliance for TB Drug Development was launched in 2000 with the goal of providing better treatment for tuberculosis by 2010 and ensuring that access to treatment is equitable. It has adopted a two-pronged R&D strategy: 1) outsourcing the development of promising anti-TB compounds to public and private collaborators worldwide, and 2) identifying and supporting projects that address critical infrastructure gaps and help to streamline the process for the successful registration of anti-TB medicines.

The Malaria Vaccine Initiative is run by an international, non-profit organization, the Program for Appropriate Technology in Health, and was established in 1999. It seeks to promote the development of promising malaria vaccines and make them more accessible in the developing world. Current projects include a deal with GlaxoSmithKline Biologicals to develop and test GSK Biologicals's malaria vaccine for children.

Five key issues have been identified that could affect the immediate and long-term credibility and performance of the PPPs described above *(2)*. Two of these issues directly concern leadership: 1) the importance of effective managers with commercial experience and good decision-makers with scientific and political experience; and 2) governance, including the choice of projects and the choice of board members. The other three issues are the strategies for the R&D process, intellectual property policies, and financial viability of the PPPs. The general conclusion is that all four partnerships have successfully initiated research programmes. The main challenge that lies ahead is whether they can continue to raise funds and secure deals with industry to meet their product and cost targets.

For more information visit the Initiative on Public-Private Partnerships for Health at: www.ippph.org

References

1. Buse K, Walt G. Global Public-Private Partnerships: Part II—What are the Health Issues for Global Governance? *Bulletin of the World Health Organization*, 2000, 78(5):699-708.
2. Kettler H, Towse A. *Public Private Partnerships for Research and Development: Medicines and Vaccines for Diseases of Poverty*, London, Office of Health Economics, 2002.

research. Part of the vision is to negotiate an acceptable balance between the goals of better health and health equity and those of economic competitiveness, market expansion and increased profits. Making explicit these differences can enhance policy discussions.

3.4 Financing: more funds or better use of existing funds?

Both are needed. In many countries, the potential for research to address and solve health problems is hampered by a lack of funds. Many national governments allocate almost none of their health budgets towards health research on a systematic basis, even if other sources of public funding may exist. The Commission on Health Research for Development recommended in its 1990 report that all countries invest at least 2% of their national health budgets in health research and building health research capacity.

Some countries and regions have since made a concerted effort to increase health research funding. For example, within India's National Health Policy of 2002, the government pledged to increase the proportion of health spending allocated to health research from 0.5% to 2% by 2010. Similarly, WHO's Eastern Mediterranean Regional Office (EMRO) recommends that member states in the region allocate 2% to 3% of the health budget to national health research systems. This was supported by a Regional Committee resolution stating that 2% of national WHO budgets should be used for health research and is currently implemented in the countries of that region.

But what amount of resources needs to be invested and should this proportion be the same in all countries? This question is more difficult to answer, given competing national priorities, differences in the organization and efficiency of health research activities, and comparative advantages in research in each country.

The Global Forum for Health Research estimated a few years ago that total funding for health research, including public, private and private non-profit funding worldwide was about US$73.5 billion or about 2.7% of total health expenditures *(6)*. Public funding represented approximately 50% of the total—or about US$37 billion in 2001—with only 3% coming from low- and middle-income countries. Increased government commitment for a systematic approach to research funding in low- and middle-income countries must be coupled with better use of existing funds.

There needs to be more transparency in the flow of health research funds. It is important to know who is funding health research, what topics and activities are being funded, and how much money is being pledged. For this reason policy discussions concerning the financing of health research must include the following three issues:

- securing research funds for the health research system;

- allocating these financial resources to projects and activities in a transparent way;
- achieving an appropriate balance between scientific curiosity and strategic needs.

Tapping into new sources of funds for health research

Policy-makers can explore a range of potential tools and approaches to increase sustainable sources of finance for health research. For example, WHO recommends earmarking a portion of tax revenue on tobacco products to fund health promotion initiatives and research. Dozens of countries target tobacco taxes to that effect. An important example is the government of Australia's Tobacco Act 1987, which created the Victorian Health Promotion Foundation (VicHealth). Originally financed from earmarked tobacco taxes, VicHealth has invested about 20% of its funds in public health research since its inception, for the equivalent of about US$70 million. VicHealth's major areas of investment include research fellowships and long-term research projects in tobacco control, mental health, physical activity, nutrition, ageing, sexually transmitted diseases, injury prevention, skin cancer prevention, and eye health.

Inspired by the Australian approach, the Thai government created the Thai Health Promotion Foundation (ThaiHealth) in 2001 which is funded from 2% of tobacco and alcohol taxes. ThaiHealth's priorities include tobacco control, alcohol control and traffic accident prevention where the production and transfer of knowledge are both key components. Other examples include Finland, which earmarks 0.45% of the estimated annual revenues from the tobacco tax for tobacco control, health education and research, and Portugal, which earmarks 1% for cancer research, prevention, diagnosis and treatment. Box 3.5 outlines innovative approaches to funding health research from Argentina and Brazil.

How to increase systematic accounting of health research flows

Some countries are already tracking their national health expenditures through a system called National Health Accounts (NHA) so that they have a clearer idea of how much funding is going into health research. This approach has been institutionalized in many countries, and covers spending on health care and health-related activities such as health research, environmental health and training of health personnel. All OECD countries, for example, compile national health accounts annually. Over 80 low- and middle-income countries have national health account estimates for at least one year.

The recording of resources invested in health systems in national health accounts is not perfect but it provides a good start and NHA has become the internationally accepted system for estimating national health expenditure. The NHA Producer's Guide is aimed at low- and middle-income countries (7) in particular and countries can use it as a tool to estimate funding flows. Demand for national health accounts has increased in recent years not least

Box 3.5 Innovative financing schemes for health research

Sao Paulo, Brazil

The Brazilian government introduced a novel scheme called sectoral funding in 1999. The aim was to increase research funding provided by the State of Sao Paulo Research Foundation (FAPESP) which already manages 1% of the state revenues for research purposes. Under this scheme, taxes from 12 sectors: oil and gas, electricity, mineral resources, water resources, space, transportation, aeronautics, health, agribusiness, biotechnology, telecommunications, and information technology and from two non-sectoral sources were funnelled into the National Fund for Science and Technology Development (FNDCT). This strategy has significantly increased the FNDCT budget from US$20 million in 1999 to US$500 million in 2002.

Argentina

In July 2003 Tulio Del Bono, Argentina's Secretary of Science, presented the parliamentary science commission in his country with three novel proposals for science and technology funding:

- A scheme known as Debt for Knowledge envisages putting 1% of the interest owed to foreign creditors into science and technology. Del Bono said this could be seen as a way of using science and technology as "motors of the country's development".
- The creation of a new risk capital fund for innovative technology companies was proposed. This envisaged an initial government investment of US$6.2 million.
- Sectoral funding based on the Brazilian programme described above under which science and technology companies would pay a tax to support research in their own areas.

Sources:
Brazil: www.fapesp.br/english
Argentina: www.scidev.net/News/index.cfm?fuseaction=readNews&itemid=934

as countries decentralize their public health services and expand coverage of national health insurance programmes. The NHA can also help countries to identify potential areas of health reform and to track the progress of reforms based on what is actually spent.

More can be done to improve the reporting of expenditure for health research in the NHA. At present health research is classified only as a health-related item in the NHA system and not considered part of the core health expenditures. Therefore, only a few countries using NHAs report health research and for those countries that do, the reported expenditure is incomplete. For example, health research expenditures by the private sector, such as pharmaceutical companies, are not included in the NHA. And some research and development activities are reported in other categories, rather than as health research.

WHO and the Global Forum for Health Research are currently working together with a range of low- and middle-income countries to develop and pilot a method for estimating resource flows for health research at the country level, based on expenditure of health research institutions. This approach will generate a more comprehensive estimate of health research funds. It will also provide information on how resources are being used in terms of the types and topics of research funded—information that is currently not available from the NHA system. One aim is to integrate the new methods tested into the NHA system, as has been done for other specialized areas within health systems—such as estimations of expenditures in reproductive health or HIV/AIDS. A successful integration would lead to a sustainable system for monitoring resource flows for health research.

3.5 Resources: people and organizations matter

A wide range of skilled individuals is critical to create research and knowledge, and to serve as a link between knowledge gained and new approaches to improve health. It is vital to get a snapshot of the national "stock" of trained and active health research workers and the "flow" of these human resources within a country or geographic region, and to other countries over a defined period of time. Such information can help develop policies and interventions to strengthen capacities.

Many ways of analysing human resources issues are commonly used in science and technology *(8)*. Selected national profiles on human resources from the Ibero-American and Inter-American Network on Science and Technology Indicators (RICYT) database illustrate some of these perspectives, and include:

- **Profile of the classes of science and innovation workers:** the mix of researchers, scholars with doctoral degrees and other research and development assistants, technicians, and other science and technology services staff found within a country (see Figure 3.5a) and the proportion of women in each class (see Figure 3.5b). For national health research systems, information on those who manage research, and synthesize, adapt and disseminate research or who integrate new knowledge within health systems would also be useful.
- **Profile of science and innovation workers in different sectors:** the mix in sectors of employment provides an understanding of the spread of human resources and potential for innovation across the economy. Four common groupings include government, business enterprise, higher education, and private non-profit sectors (see Figure 3.5c). Also informative for national

Figure 3.5a Percentage of researchers by types of science and technology personnel in selected Latin American countries

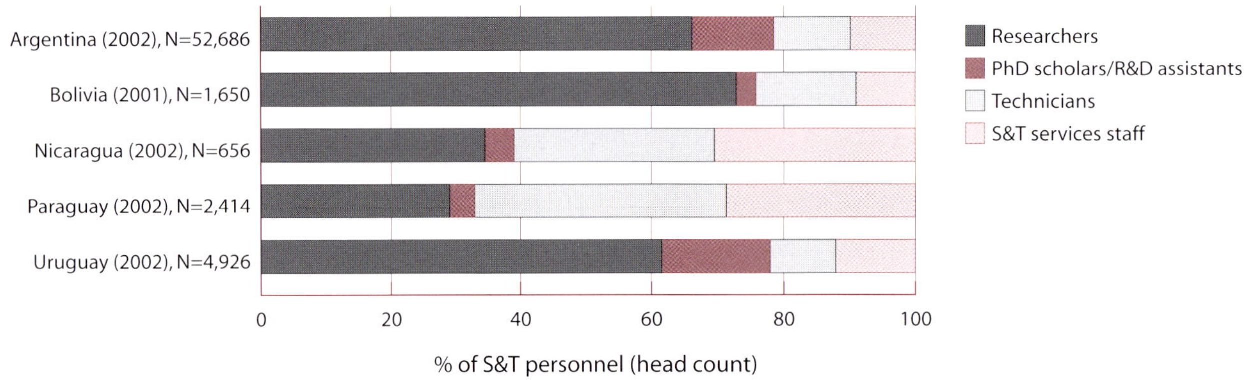

Source: Selected countries from the Ibero American Network on Science and Technology Indicators (RICYT) database, year of data indicated for each country.

health research systems would be workers in international organizations located in the country and the rest of the world. The so-called "diaspora" refers to citizens of countries who work in another country. For example, they might be on secondment, or commuting regularly across national

Figure 3.5b Proportion of women within each class of science and technology personnel in selected Latin American countries

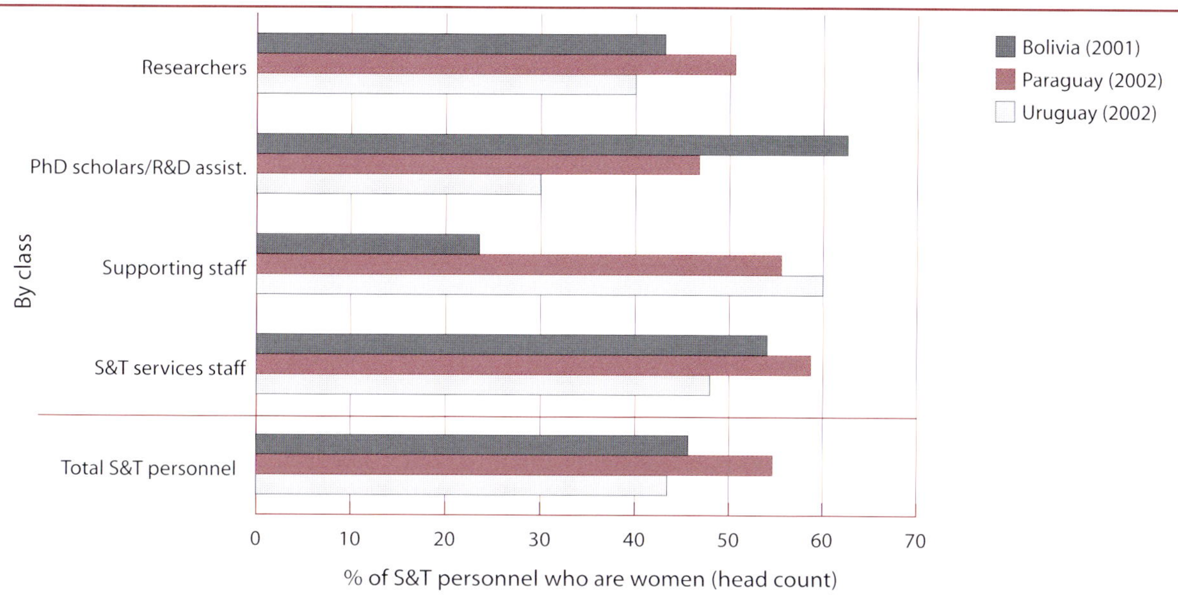

Source: Selected countries from the Ibero American Network on Science and Technology Indicators (RICYT) database, year of data indicated for each country.

Figure 3.5c Percentage of researchers by sector of employment in selected Latin American countries compared to the USA

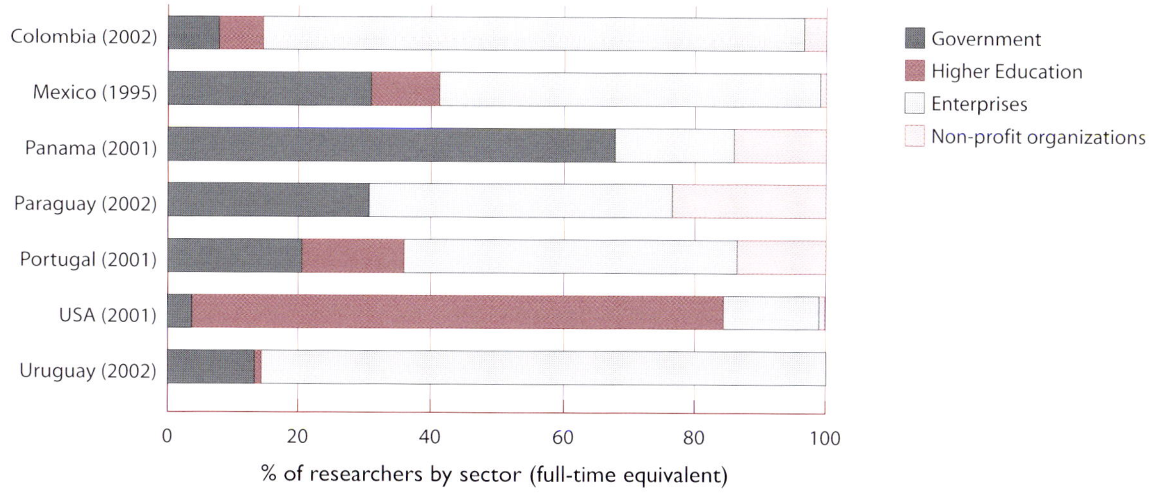

Source: Selected countries from the Ibero American Network on Science and Technology Indicators (RICYT) database, year of data indicated for each country.

borders or working abroad on a more permanent basis but maintaining close links with home-based institutions. By one estimate, 80% of foreign students from China and India planned to stay in the United States on completion of their studies; 60% of them had definite job offers *(9)*.

- **Profile of science and technology workers by different fields of science**: the mix of researchers addressing six major fields of science (see Figure 3.5d). For national health research systems, more detailed information on disciplines and fields that are relevant to health and health system challenges would be useful for planning purposes.

Medical and health research councils across South Asia have noted that there is a lack of expertise in health economics, epidemiology, anthropology and health policy *(10)*. This is coupled with a shortage of staff with statistical, analytical and managerial skills. Limited capacities in these areas have severely reduced the ability to translate questions asked by policy-makers into research questions with appropriate methodologies, develop comprehensive research proposals or oversee complex research projects. What is also important is that these skills are also relevant to functions that need to be upgraded within the region's national health systems: disease surveillance, health and management information systems, quality assurance activities or vital registration systems.

It is necessary to find other ways to strengthen existing capacities or build up capacities in less developed areas. These should be tailored to each country, taking stock of reviews for capacity-building approaches from other countries (see Box 3.6 for an example from South Africa).

Health research priorities and human resources capacities differ from country to country. It is not surprising that there is much debate on whose capacities should be strengthened. Should it be traditional researchers, health

Figure 3.5d Percentage of science and technology personnel by field of science in selected Latin American countries

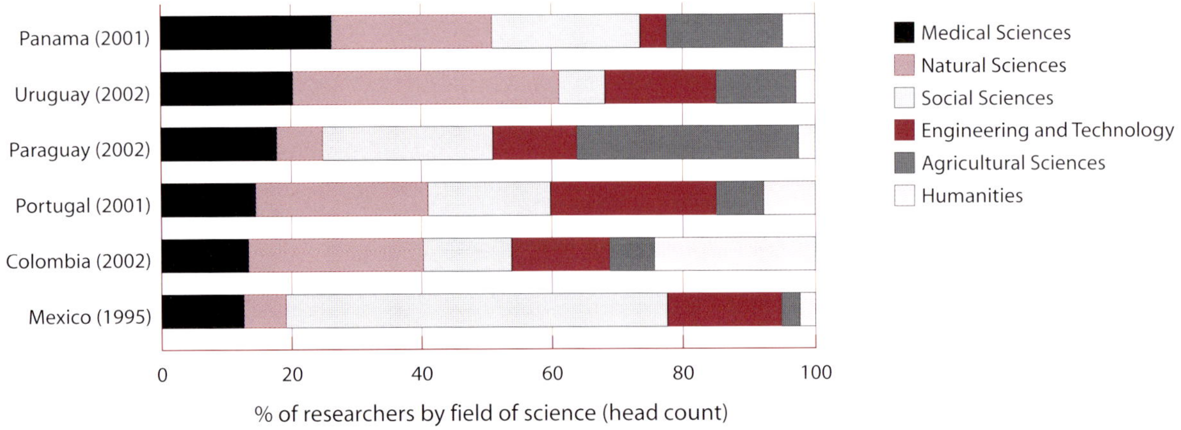

Source: Selected countries from the Ibero American Network on Science and Technology Indicators (RICYT) database, year of data indicated for each country

Box 3.6 Building research capacity in South Africa

The South African National Department of Health, supported by South Africa's Essential National Health Research Committee, recently funded a review of health research capacity building in the country. It investigated a range of informal and formal health research capacity building initiatives in South Africa. The informal initiatives are those involving employees of the public health system—part of the non-traditional researcher community—in conducting research. It also included a review of initiatives that have been sponsored by international organizations or others outside the country, and discussed the implications for South Africa. Several key factors considered necessary for the success of research capacity building initiatives were identified:

- Pursuing higher qualifications, particularly doctoral degrees, as a means to further develop independent thinking and increase productivity.
- Collaborating with other research programmes to further promote a culture of writing, of compiling statistical analyses and of using databases. This might involve mentoring by senior researchers and collaboration between experienced and inexperienced people to increase confidence.
- Capacity building for skills that are relevant to local priorities and the health development needs of the country increases the likelihood that research results are used.
- Recognizing that developing research skills takes time and commitment so researchers should be involved in fields that interest them and where they can have influence.
- Recruiting motivated individuals as well as those with persistence, initiative and concern to improve public health.

Source: *Health Research Capacity Building in South Africa: current knowledge and practices.* Durban, Health Systems Trust, 2003.

services professionals, social scientists, or local health workers? Where and what type of training should be offered, and to what extent should capacity strengthening activities be integrated within "hands-on" research activities? Furthermore, many capacity strengthening activities are informal, often based on personal contacts developed through professional groups or collaboration among institutions.

How much should be spent on capacity strengthening within national health research systems? The Commission on Health Research and Development suggested in 1990 that international donors including aid agencies should commit at least 5% of health project aid for essential national health research and research capacity building. In a study of more than 3,000 people working in national health research systems in 13 low- and middle-income countries, respondents said that of the total financial resources devoted to health research, approximately 82% should be spent on research activities covering fundamental research, health conditions, risk factors, or health systems research. The balance should be spent on capacity building for health research to best achieve national health research priorities.

It also seems that some funders of capacity building initiatives focus on a relatively narrow range of traditional activities, whereas many successful projects and interventions also promote more innovative or experimental initiatives and partnerships. For example, in the area of technology transfers in biomedical and vaccine research, partnerships on the international and regional scale have forged successful approaches (see Box 3.7). This is yet another example of international strategic research.

Fostering an enabling environment for producing research

In addition to strengthening human capacity, efforts must be made by countries to foster a supportive working environment for researchers (see Box 3.8).

Box 3.7 Technology transfer to developing countries

Sustainable Sciences Institute

The Sustainable Sciences Institute (SSI) is a non-profit organization based in San Francisco in the United States that helps scientists in developing countries gain access to the resources needed to address local problems related to infectious diseases.

Dr Eva Harris and her colleagues at SSI have demonstrated by transferring technologies and adapting these to local conditions in developing countries, sophisticated molecular biology methods which were previously unattainable can contribute to the education, health and human rights of the population.

As part of its technology transfer programmes, SSI runs workshops to introduce researchers mainly from Latin American countries to the techniques of molecular biology, epidemiology and scientific writing. The aim is to sharpen the researchers' ability to initiate independent research. The workshops also adapt biomedical techniques to local research priorities and conditions to help countries build the necessary capability to conduct locally relevant research. This is an essential prerequisite for the development of public health programmes. These workshops address some of the major barriers faced, including limited access to technologies, scientific isolation, a lack of information and the absence of technical training programmes and scientific career opportunities. The SSI workshops have been held in 12 countries in Latin America as well as in Egypt, sparking collaborative projects, locally funded proposals and scientific publications. So far, SSI has trained more than 600 scientists and health professionals in 20 developing countries.

SSI also runs a small-grants programme that funds some of the best proposals generated during the workshops. In addition, SSI facilitates the donation of scientific equipment and supplies from biotech companies and university laboratories in developed countries to trainee researchers in the developed world.

These programmes show that molecular technologies can be adapted to local conditions and disease priorities in developing countries to be more rapid, versatile, and sensitive than alternative methods. These methods can be cost-effective in low-budget situations, as demonstrated through the work of Bolivian investigator Nataniel Mamani, who created the blenderfuge. This combines a blender, an aluminium bowl and water-tap adapters to create a microcentrifuge, and the turntable shaker, where the circular rotation of a record player is transformed into a horizontal shaker for the laboratory.

For more information visit: www.ssilink.org

A record player turntable becomes a laboratory shaker

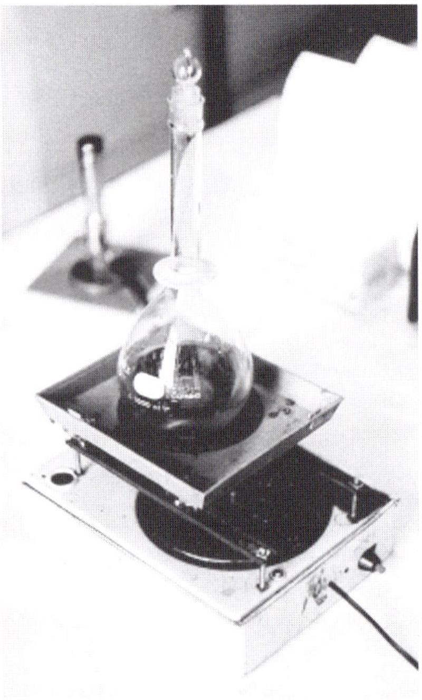

Photo by Nataniel Mamani, Universidad Mayor de San Andrés, La Paz, Bolivia.

Source: Harris E, Tanner M. Health technology transfer. *British Medical Journal*, 2000, 321:817–820.

continued

Research has shown that pay is not the only concern of those within health research systems. According to data from across 13 low- and middle-income countries, those surveyed within national health research systems ranked transparency of the funding process before salary and benefits. They said these were the most important areas for further strengthening, followed by quality of the work space and facilities, training and ongoing training opportunities.

These areas for strengthening require a change in attitudes and a more performance-oriented culture, not just financial resources. This includes a change in the management and organization of research institutions, as well as a change in social attitudes towards research and health research in particular. For example, the social status attached to research and researchers varies greatly by scientific field, common methods used, institutional ties, or relevance to social problems as well as in relation to other professions. To produce and

Box 3.7 Technology transfer to developing countries *(continued)*

Meningitis Vaccine Project

The Meningitis Vaccine Project (MVP), a partnership between the WHO and the Program for Appropriate Technology in Health (PATH), seeks to develop meningococcal conjugate vaccines for use in Africa (www.meningvax.org). When looking for a partner, MVP decided against an established vaccine manufacturer in an industrialized country. Instead, it opted to transfer technology to a manufacturer in a developing country (see figure). The reason was that the manufacturer in the industrialized country viewed factors such as: capital investment for vaccine production, selling vaccines to Africa with a low profit margin and acquiring capacity that could be used to create other vaccines for profit as expensive. In contrast, the manufacturer in the developing country saw these as opportunities. By working with a manufacturer in a developing country, the vaccine would be developed as a high-priority product specifically for use in Africa rather than an adapted version of a vaccine developed for other markets (and possibly different strains). In early 2004, PATH entered into a long-term sub-license and supply agreement with the Serum Institute of India based in the Indian city of Pune to develop, test and produce clinical and commercial lots of group A meningococcal conjugate vaccine. The Phase I trial of this vaccine was due to begin by January 2005. The vaccine has a target price of US$0.40 per dose, one fifth of the cost of similar vaccines developed in the West.

MVP's alternative approaches to vaccine development

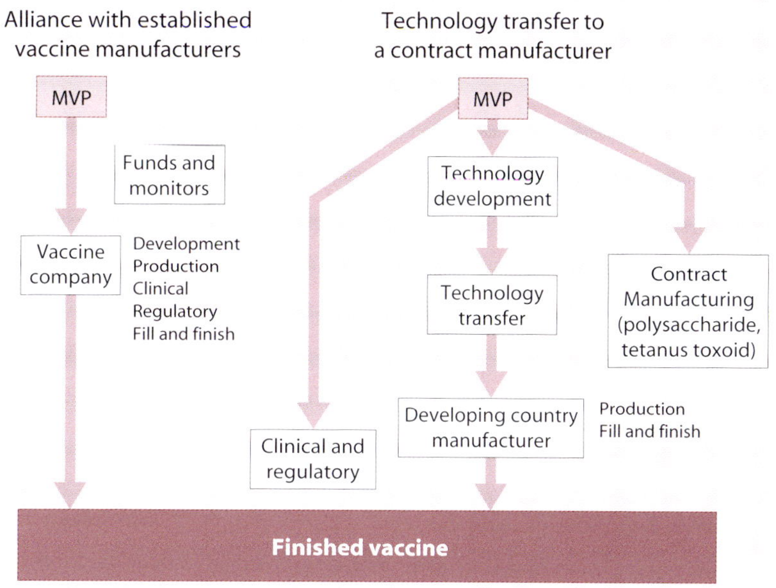

For more information visit: www.meningvax.org

Source: Jódar L et al. Meningococcal conjugate vaccine for Africa: a model for development of new vaccines for the poorest countries. *Lancet*, 2003, 361:1902–1904.

use knowledge for better health, the national health research system should develop approaches to put greater value on the social science disciplines (e.g. economics, demography, sociology, anthropology, and others), non-traditional research methods, and locations of research that have greater interface with the health system.

Studies *(11)* have shown that factors that contribute to migration of health researchers (and other health professionals) in many low-income countries include poor career opportunities at home (see Box 3.9). Information on the migration of health professionals, particularly doctors and nurses, for some countries, is becoming more available, yet there is almost no data specific to the migration of health researchers.

Promoting collaboration in health research

One option for countries to strengthen research capacity is to increase health research collaboration between institutions, within countries as well as across national borders. Based on experiences from China and India, this is one

Box 3.8 Creating an enabling working environment

Several low- and middle-income countries helped to identify 10 key areas that need to be addressed to create an enabling environment for health research workers. These emerged in a series of discussions as part of the WHO-sponsored health research systems analysis project. These areas relate to science, education and health systems:

Range and breadth of health researchers: establish teams of researchers who have a range of experiences and skills and who work in a variety of health research disciplines, from basic science to health systems and social science to epidemiology.

Transparency of the funding process: adopt a merit-based, accountable funding procedure with clear criteria and prompt processing.

Quality of workspace and facilities: provide functional workspaces with access to relevant technologies and materials.

Encouragement of collaboration with others: promote collaboration both home and abroad among researchers as well as among researchers, health professionals, policy-makers, the media, civil society and the public.

Opportunities to present, discuss, and publish results: provide opportunities and incentives to discuss and present both work in progress and completed, as well as publish results in a diverse range of journals or other media. Opportunities to participate in international conferences are particularly important.

Relevance of health research activities to health problems and health systems: address priority areas of research, current or projected health problems, and health problems of disadvantaged or poor populations, both at national and global levels.

Remuneration of health researchers: provide adequate salary and benefits to recruit and retain trained health researchers.

Nurturing of careers: recognize work contribution and provide mentoring and leadership opportunities for young and mid-level researchers.

Training and ongoing training: provide up-to-date training on the latest conceptual, methodological and technical advances in health research and establish a continuous education programme.

Access and sharing of information: ensure access to national, regional, and international publications, electronic information sources, and reference databases on a range of health research disciplines.

These research findings show that the chief concern of people working in the health research sector is not primarily pay. Health research workers surveyed in 13 low- and middle-income countries, ranked transparency of the funding process as one of the most important areas for further strengthening of the health research system. This was followed by quality of work space, facilities and training.

Source: Health Research Systems Analyses Initiative, World Health Organization.

way of maintaining productive ties between researchers who have migrated to other countries. More collaboration in health research would increase the flow of knowledge between researchers by bringing together people, ideas and technologies. Moreover, many national and regional science policies would benefit from greater integration in regional or international activities. For smaller countries or those with more limited research capacities, collaboration can be a powerful approach to gain access to external resources and reach a wider audience.

For example, collaboration patterns across institutions and countries can be estimated from international reference databases of research outputs if addresses of all co-authors are included. Based on articles addressing health topics in peer reviewed journals included within the Thomson ISI databases during 2001, Figure 3.6 provides the number of papers with at least one co-author from each of WHO's geographic regions.

Collaborations within a single institution, or across institutions within the same country, make up the largest portion of articles for countries with a relatively developed health research system. Less developed countries tend to have more international collaboration. Drawing from a survey of more

Box 3.9 Brain drain or science gain?

The migration of scientists presents a growing challenge for policy-makers in many developing countries as borders become increasingly fluid. According to a recent report from the French development agency Institut de recherche pour le développement (IRD), "roughly one-third of the total scientific and technical community of the Southern countries are working in the North," and two-thirds of Southern expatriate students settle permanently in their host countries.

There are many factors driving scientists out of lower-income countries: low salaries; poor equipment and working conditions; lack of academic liberty and incentives to sustain research efforts; inadequate educational systems; failing economies; high unemployment rates; inadequate social services; excessive bureaucracy; oppressive political environments; discrimination and armed conflict

At the same time, higher-income countries have a growing demand for skilled professionals and offer many benefits such as: attractive pay packages, policies to ease visa applications, high standard of living, pensions, educational and career opportunities, and professional recognition.

Some view this as a brain drain particularly where the migration of health professionals may cause serious deficiencies in national health research, access and coverage. "The cost of training is borne by the poor country and the rich country reaps the benefits," Vikram Patel wrote in the *British Medical Journal* in October 2003.

Others view this more as "brain circulation", such as Jean-Baptiste Meyer from France's Institut de recherche pour le développement who wrote in an article on web-based health information service SciDevNet in May 2003: "The mobility of highly skilled manpower should be seen as a normal process that should not be stopped, and the real challenge is therefore to manage it as well as possible".

Policy options

Countries have taken various measures to address staff shortages resulting from the migration of health researchers. Wisdom J. Tettey, professor at the Faculty of Communication and Culture of the University of Calgary, Canada, noted in an article in *SciDevNet* in May 2003 that some African countries, including South Africa, Senegal, Tanzania, Egypt, and Morocco, had national research grant schemes for professionals to pursue careers in their chosen field without having to leave the country.

"Establishment of endowed chairs—through state, private, bilateral, or multilateral partnerships—can also help to keep some top African experts in their countries, and even attract those currently elsewhere," Tettey concluded.

Robyn Iredale, associate professor at the School of Geosciences of the University of Wollongong in Australia wrote in an article in *SciDevNet* in August 2003 that the former Committee on Science and Technology in Developing Countries of the International Council for Science had proposed the establishment of an Intellectual Resources Management Fund to address losses from brain drain and improve the standards of science and technology professionals.

"Monies collected from receiving countries that benefit from skilled immigration would be used towards additional training, exchanges and collaboration, and better working conditions in the developing world," Iredale said.

Jacques Gaillard, deputy director of the International Foundation for Science in Sweden and social anthropologist Anne Marie Gaillard write about another initiative to turn the brain drain into a chance for technology transfer.

In *SciDevNet* in May 2003 they wrote that the New Partnership for Africa's Development (NEPAD) seems to endorse the "scientific diaspora option" by calling for the development of "scientific and technical networks to channel the repatriation of scientific knowledge to the home country, and establish co-operation between those abroad and at home."

They argued that the diaspora model, however, would never be a low-cost, self-sufficient answer to Africa's scientific needs because its effectiveness depends on the internal dynamics of the home-based scientific communities.

"After all, a network of expatriates is at best an extension of a national scientific community, not a substitute. Efforts should therefore, first and foremost, focus on strengthening national scientific capacity particularly training and recruiting the next generation of scientists," they wrote.

For more information visit: Institut de recherche pour le développement (IRD) : www.ird.fr

Source: Patel V. Recruiting doctors from poor countries: the great brain robbery? *British Medical Journal*, 2003, 327: 926–928.

than 3,000 individuals within national health research systems in 13 low- and middle-income countries, collaboration within countries is concentrated among academic and research institutions, university hospitals and national ministries of health. Significantly less collaboration is reported with patient and consumer groups, national technical and regulatory agencies, or alternative health-care providers (*12*).

Existing approaches to strengthen research collaboration span a wide range of activities, from sharing experiences and facilitating discussions at regular gatherings, to supporting cross-institutional and cross-border training

Figure 3.6 Collaboration in health research production for WHO Regions, 2001

	Number of papers from Thomson ISI database						
WHO Region	*AFRO*	*AMRO*	*EMRO*	*EURO*	*SEARO*	*WPRO*	*Total*
AFRO	1,298	—	—	—	—	—	2,843
AMRO	589	119,750	—	—	—	—	144,755
EMRO	28	331	2,057	—	—	—	2,940
EURO	1,104	18,313	541	120,361	—	—	143,758
SEARO	25	596	41	523	3,885	—	5,175
WPRO	160	6,807	93	4,558	365	43,502	54,115

Note: The total number of papers for a region/country may not be equal to the sum of papers written in collaboration with regions, as some papers may be written in collaboration with more than one region/country.

WHO Regional Offices:

AFRO: WHO Regional Office for Africa
AMRO: WHO Regional Office for the Americas
EMRO: WHO Regional Office for the Eastern Mediterranean
EURO: WHO Regional Office for Europe
SEARO: WHO Regional Office for South-East Asia
WPRO: WHO Regional Office for the Western Pacific

Source: Health Research Systems Analyses Initiative estimations based on Thomson ISI Web of Science database, World Health Organization.

schemes. Box 3.10 shows three notable examples of cross-national collaboration initiatives and networks, from the Pasteur Institute, the Special Programme on Tropical Diseases Research (TDR) and Special Programme of Research, Development and Research Training in Human Reproduction (HRP).

3.6 Producing, synthesizing, and using research

Are the products of research being used?

As noted in Section 3.1, there is a wide range of research outputs including scientific publications, policy publications, reports, books, discussion papers and patents. The fourth function of a health research system is not only to produce research but also to use research to improve health.

Research can be used in several ways: for developing new interventions (drugs, vaccines, devices and other applications) to improve health; and for translating, communicating, and promoting the use of research to inform health policies, strategies, and practices, particularly within health systems (see Chapter 4). Research can also be used to inform the population and change public opinion and practices.

Yet one major deficiency in health research systems across countries is that the research process and the policy process tend to exist in different worlds. The result is that research often has limited relevance to or impact on policy. It is also well recognized that much of public health decision-making and public health practices are neither based on evidence nor evaluated for effectiveness, efficiency, or equity. One of the major causes of this gap is the inability to

Box 3.10 Fostering international collaboration

The Pasteur Institute

The Pasteur Institute is a private, non-profit foundation whose mission is to prevent and treat health conditions, particularly infectious diseases, through biological research, training and application to public health.

This foundation has an extensive international network composed of 25 independent Pasteur Institutes across the world (see map below). In addition to conducting scientific research, these provide services such as testing vaccines, training staff and external scientific researchers and they are involved in public health activities, with eight branches serving as WHO collaborating centres.

The Pasteur Institute also has an International Affairs division which seeks to promote collaboration in scientific research on a regional and global level. The division has several international collaboration initiatives (see map below) in the form of scientific partnerships, foundations or associations. An example of a regional scientific partnership is Amsud, which is composed of the Mercosur countries: Argentina, Brazil, Uruguay, and Paraguay, plus Chile.

For more information about the Pasteur Institute and its activities, visit: www.pasteur.fr

Centres that collaborate with or are part of the Pasteur Institute

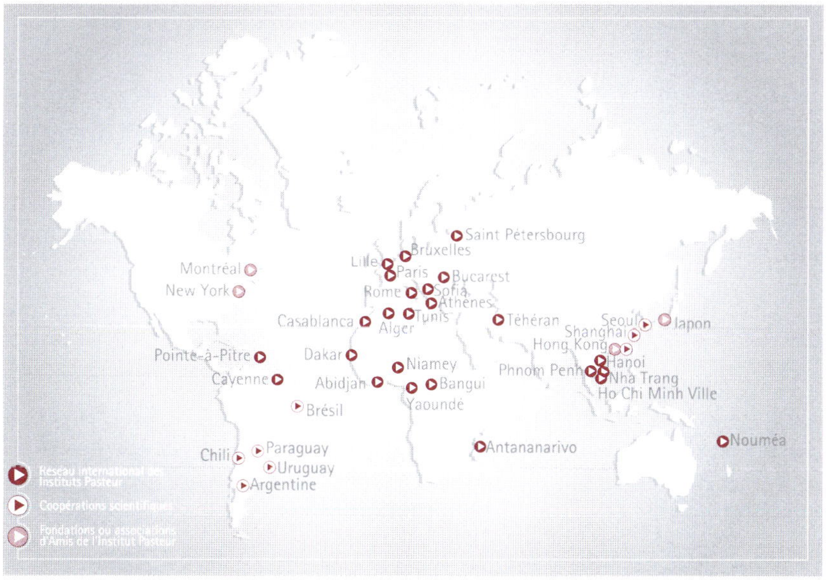

Special Programme for Research and Training in Tropical Diseases (TDR)

The Special Programme for Research and Training in Tropical Diseases (TDR) is an independent programme of scientific collaboration, co-sponsored by the United Nations Children's Fund (UNICEF), the United Nations Development Programme (UNDP), the World Bank and WHO. This programme aims to improve research and development in neglected infectious diseases and strengthen capacity in developing countries to enable them to carry out the research needed to develop and implement disease control measures.

Known as the Tropical Disease Research programme or TDR, this initiative provides direction and grants for research priorities, opportunities and training. It has formed research partnerships with several organizations, including national governments, research institutions, disease control programmes, NGOs, industry and academia. It has also supported capacity building efforts in over 400 institutions in about 80 countries.

Through its co-sponsors and networks that span many disciplines and sectors, the TDR programme provides technical expertise in a wide range of research in tropical diseases, from biomedical science and product development to more applied research such as clinical field research, capacity building and communication.

For more information about the TDR programme, visit: www.who.int/tdr

UNDP/UNFPA/WHO/World Bank Special Programme of Research, Development and Research Training in Human Reproduction (HRP)

The Human Reproduction Programme's mission is to help developing countries develop and implement national and regional research findings as well as programmes aimed at improving reproductive health. HRP seeks to review, develop and test methodologies for the planning and implementation of reproductive health services, and to provide technical support to assist countries to do so. Central to this are efforts to refine, promote and assist countries in implementation of the Strategic Approach, a set of guidelines agreed by the partners in the project, to promote reproductive health policy and programme development. Other activities related to HRP are highlighted in Boxes 3.13 and 4.10.

For more information about HRP visit: www.who.int/reproductive-health/hrp/index.html

synthesize existing research outputs and apply existing knowledge towards improving interventions and the performance of health systems. Gathering this evidence and knowledge for improving health is precisely one role of health systems and health policy research.

The process of conducting research studies and utilizing knowledge is a highly complex one. Far greater use must be made of systematic reviews that attempt to distil and synthesize the vast amount of research results in a manner that will help to inform researchers, policy-makers, practitioners, and members of the public. These research syntheses are important because of the cumulative nature of science, the knowledge "explosion", and haphazard and biased publication or access to research (see also Section 1.5).

The impact of research on public opinion is receiving increasing attention, with particular interest in novel communication and dissemination approaches as a means of increasing public awareness and understanding, as well as the relevance of research results. But much more progress is needed. In a recent review of some 40 major newspapers across 13 low- and middle-income countries, it was found that very few articles on health research gave credit to the policies and activities that have allowed research to take place, or how new discoveries build on existing knowledge *(12)*. Even fewer articles discuss how the new knowledge may be applied within health systems, for example to improve services to vulnerable groups or the public at large.

Active two-way engagement between the community and the health research system is seen to be increasingly important, with some communities and patient groups getting involved in guiding research priorities and participating in the conduct of research. Such involvement would help to ensure the effective application of research findings.

Finding the right balance

In terms of the production and use of research, a global health research system has to attempt to find a balance between three areas: (1) producing scientifically valid fundamental research outputs; (2) promoting the use of research to develop drugs, vaccines, devices and other applications to improve health; (3) translating, synthesizing and communicating research to inform health policy, health practice and public opinion *(13)*. In most countries much of the emphasis is on the first, with some on the second, and almost none on the third. Articles addressing public health remain a low proportion of papers published in peer reviewed journals that are shared in international databases (see Figure 3.7). Moreover, less than a tenth of the Cochrane Collaboration's reviews are on public health interventions. This low proportion is perhaps a key reason that led the Cochrane Collaboration to set up a "Health Promotion and Public Health Field" to improve the relevance of its systematic reviews to global public health priorities *(14)*.

In addition, the research base addressing diseases that have the greatest burden is extremely thin. Systematic reviews are impossible if there are not enough articles to be synthesized. For instance, Figure 3.8 illustrates that systematic reviews on child health include almost no studies on the effectiveness of health interventions. With so few studies addressing interventions for populations in greatest need, it is difficult to develop evidence-based policies.

The challenge facing governments, the international community and an

Figure 3.7 Publications in journals addressing health topics by field, 1992–2001

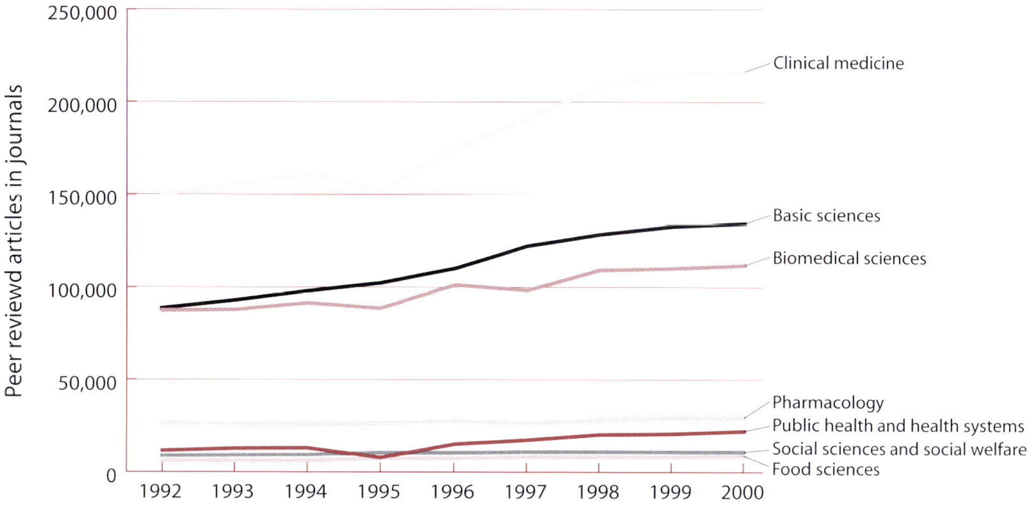

Note: Journals are classified based on Thomson ISI categories and own selection of journals addressing broad range of health topics.

Source: Health Research Systems Analyses estimations based on Thomson ISI database 2001.

Figure 3.8 Analysis of systematic reviews for selected health interventions

Proportion and topic of research articles included within systematic research syntheses addressing diarrhoea, acute respiratory infections (ARI), micronutrient deficiencies and neonatal disorders

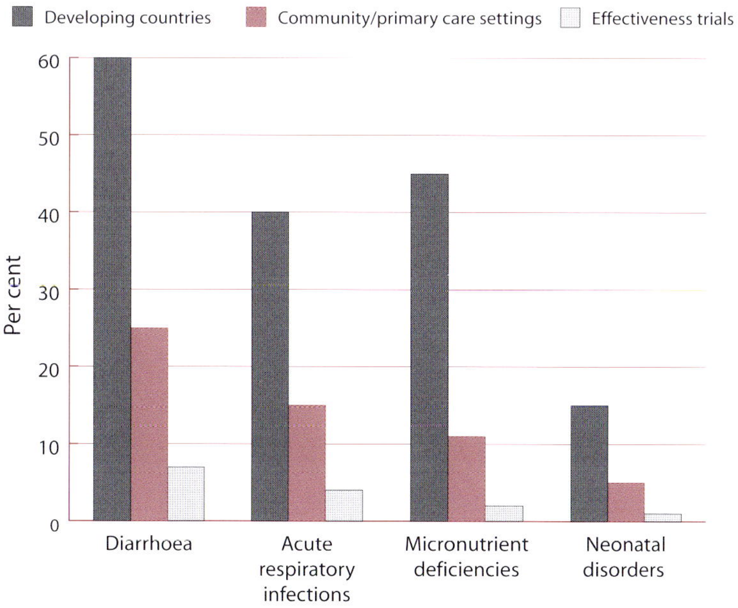

Source: Bhutta et al. (2004, unpublished)

increasingly engaged public is to create an environment in which evidence is routinely used in health systems decision-making. It is with this perspective that one should understand the production and use of research in countries. With this in mind, WHO is working with 10 low- and middle-income countries to examine how research is used as an input to decision-making. Some of the specific topics include the prevention of malaria, oral rehydration therapy (ORT), DOTS strategy for tuberculosis control, and contraceptive method mix to increase women's choices for birth control. This project is being done with support from the Global Development Network and the Alliance for Health Policy and Systems Research. The results will be used to identify interventions to increase the use of research in decision-making.

Improving access to information

All these issues surrounding the use of research and improving communication among researchers, policy-makers, and consumers are discussed in more detail in Chapter 4. But before there can be any discussion about how to better share and use research, both the producers and users of research (i.e. the public, civil society/NGOs, patients, health professionals, health system managers, health insurers, the biomedical industry, and policy-makers) must be able to access information.

In recent years there have been some moves to dismantle some of the barriers to accessing research information. Recognizing that few researchers in developing countries can afford the high cost of journal subscriptions, several initiatives have been implemented using Internet gateways to give researchers free online access to the full text of health research papers published in journals. BIREME (serving researchers in Latin America and the Caribbean) was the first and is now one of the largest sources of such information (through the Scientific Electronic Library Online or SciELO). The Ptolemy project is helping to meet the information needs of researchers in Africa. HINARI (Health InterNetwork Access to Research Initiative), a partnership led by WHO involving more than 50 international publishers, Yale University and the National Library of Medicine, is another example (see Box 3.11). HINARI has been running since January 2002 and as of mid-2004 was offering researchers in 113 developing countries online access to nearly 2,400 journals.

Another opportunity to improve access to research may come from the "open access" movement, a global initiative that is challenging the traditional subscription-based model of journals. Open access is promoting an "author-pays" model where the author is charged a fee to recover the costs associated with peer review, production, and provision of an electronic article. In reality, however, the researcher's institution or funder will usually pay the charge in order to ensure wide dissemination of the research they have supported. The final paper is available free of charge via the Internet to anyone who wants to use it. Public Library of Science (PLoS) in the United States and BioMed Central in the United Kingdom are two examples of such initiatives.

Although systematic reviews often provide the most reliable evidence about

Box 3.11 A new social contract: HINARI bridges the digital divide

Until recently, health researchers at the University of Yaounde I in Cameroon could not afford to subscribe to medical journals. Today they can download full-text articles from thousands of journals through the WHO's Health InterNetwork Access to Research initiative, better known as HINARI.

"We cannot find the words to express our satisfaction.... More than 10 years ago, we did not receive budget to acquire journals. And a few minutes ago we became rich by becoming part of HINARI," said Elisabeth Andong, from the University of Yaounde I in Cameroon, in a note of thanks to WHO.

Launched in 2002, HINARI is a WHO initiative that gives researchers, primary healthcare workers and health policy managers in developing countries free or low-cost access to a vast collection of medical journals online. Last year HINARI members downloaded more than one million articles. The HINARI database is only available in countries where the annual gross national product (GNP) per capita is less than US$3,000 per year. Ethiopia, for example, is one of the countries where HINARI is used most.

HINARI offers full-text resources to a wide range of biomedical research institutions, professional schools (medicine, nursing, pharmacy, public health, dentistry), teaching hospitals, research organizations, national universities, national medical libraries and government health ministries. All staff members and students have access to more than 2,400 journals from approximately 50 publishers—perhaps one of the most comprehensive online collections in the world—as well as access to PubMed (Medline) through the National Library of Medicine. More than 1,200 institutions in 103 out of the 113 eligible countries use HINARI.

The project started as a collaborative effort between the WHO and the British Medical Journal. The two identified six publishers who were willing to offer all of their medical information on health care as well as in primary research to institutions in the developing world. Most importantly, the six publishers: Blackwell Publishing, Elsevier, Harcourt Worldwide STM Group, Wolters Kluwer International Health & Science, Springer Verlag and John Wiley & Sons, agreed to provide online resources free of charge or at a very low cost. Yale University Library, another valuable partner in the project, offers not only the user identification system but also assistance in linking users and publishers.

"This project has probably had the most impact of any WHO project since the Oral Rehydration Therapy," said Dr Philip Njemanze, chairman of the International Institutes of Advanced Research and Training at the Chidicon Medical Center in Imo State, Nigeria." It will have the most impact on the health of the developing world," Dr Njemanze said, adding that this had enabled his own institution to triple its literature base.

For the first time, everyone from physicians, surgeons, and dentists to pharmacists, veterinarians, biologists, and chemists now have access to extremely valuable and otherwise expensive health-care information.

"It has been a very popular initiative here," said Warren Stevens of MRC Laboratories in The Gambia, adding: "Intellectual isolation is considered one of the factors African research centres cannot develop world class researchers. This can go some way to changing that."

Although HINARI is technically simple and offers authenticated users a simple gateway to their journal of interest, the problem is that many institutions in the developing world cannot afford an Internet connection or do not have a computer. A formal evaluation of HINARI will begin in 2005.

For more information visit: www.healthinternetwork.org

the effects of health-care interventions, the evidence must be made available, in an accessible form, to health-care decision-makers who have completely different information needs. They rarely access original research papers and policy-makers, for example, prefer a very concise assessment of the potential benefits of a course of action weighed against the potential harm and costs. They also want to know the applicability across groups. Some initiatives have recently been launched to meet the health information needs of those outside the research community (see Box 3.12).

Unfortunately, the digital divide in Internet access means that many people cannot benefit from these kinds of initiatives. Even when a computer is available, the cost of accessing information through the Internet remains beyond the reach of the majority of people living in developing countries. Therefore, the CD-ROM format may be the ideal platform in the short-to-medium term for material directed towards health workers. This is the approach that has been

Box 3.12 WHO's Health Evidence Network

WHO launched an information service this year called Health Evidence Network (HEN) to provide policy-makers in the WHO European Region with the evidence they need to make key decisions on health.

"Our ambition is to provide each country in the region with analysis and information that is useful to decision-makers in Member States," said Dr Marc Danzon, WHO Regional Director for Europe. The network has two services: it provides a single point for easy access to relevant evidence and information, and it provides answers to questions to support the decision-making process.

In response to policy-makers' questions, HEN identifies and reviews relevant online resources and selects information related to public health such as publications in databases and from networks of experts.

HEN's answers to these requests are based on careful reviews of scientific evidence and other relevant information. HEN provides information on what is and is not known about the issue as well as the current debate on the subject and finally sets out the policy options. This gives policy-makers a quick way to obtain evidence to back up their decisions.

HEN is advised by an international Editorial Board to ensure that the information it provides is reliable, up-to-date and relevant. The network's information is also dependent on that of partner institutions. That means, for instance, that HEN may map out online resources available from partners, which includes a content summary to show available public health evidence. With the help of the Editorial Board, HEN reviews questions posed by European health-care policy-makers and chooses which ones to respond to. Experts are then commissioned to produce evidence-based, peer reviewed and concise responses, which are occasionally updated. Examples of questions answered by HEN include:

- What are the palliative care needs of older people and how might they be met?
- How effective are mental health services for the elderly?
- What are the best strategies for ensuring quality in hospitals?

The HEN web site also facilitates access to online resources, both publishing the reports and strengthening the network of collaborating agencies.

HEN currently works with more than 30 agencies and institutions in public health, all of which contribute by proposing questions and suggesting experts who can respond to them.

For more information visit: www.euro.who.int/HEN

Box 3.13 Essential evidence for better practice in reproductive health

The WHO Reproductive Health Library (RHL) is an example of a multifaceted dissemination strategy aimed at health workers. RHL is published annually on CD-ROM in English and Spanish and is currently in its seventh edition. This CD-ROM contains a specialist database providing systematic reviews of interventions in the field of reproductive health with commentaries from people with knowledge of how these can be applied in resource-poor settings.

RHL is a collaborative effort between the WHO's Department of Reproductive Health and Research, the Cochrane Collaboration, and Reproductive Health Library partner institutions in low- and middle-income countries.

Each issue includes editorials, systematic reviews, commentaries, practical aspects documents, audio-visual aids (video clips) to assist in implementing practices, methodology papers, Internet links, list of NGOs active in reproductive health, register of donor agencies for reproductive health. Every year new content is added and about a third of evidence that has already been included is revised. In 2003 some 32,000 CD-ROMs were produced and made available free of charge to health workers in developing countries.

The WHO Department of Reproductive Health and Research has built up a subscriber base of more than 13,000 users, mostly in developing countries. In addition, an editorial team comprising seven country-based editors and the WHO secretariat regularly conducts presentations and workshops around the world. These workshops are often linked to regional or national conferences and are designed to demonstrate the use of RHL as well as giving basic training in reading and appraising synthesized evidence on reproduction issues.

WHO has developed a formal four-day training course in evidence-based decision-making in the African Region. Similar strategies combining introductory workshops with interactive educational activities are also conducted in Asia and Latin America. A randomized controlled trial evaluating an interactive educational workshop programme is currently being conducted in 22 hospitals in Mexico and 18 hospitals in Thailand. The trial aims to assess improvements in obstetric practices as a result staff being trained to use evidence presented in the Reproductive Health Library.

For more information visit: www.rhlibrary.org

adopted by WHO's Reproductive Health Library (see Box 3.13).

Wi-Fi, the wireless standard of communication also known as 802.11, is another promising technology for reaching isolated villages with minimal need for infrastructure in terms of telephones and electricity. Wi-Fi relies on inexpensive antennas rather than costly cables and receivers and may yet prove to be the answer to cheap and reliable Internet and email access (see Figure 3.9).

Regional perspective 5

Research into ways to improve knowledge transfer and access in health systems should be a priority—it should address the major barriers of financial constraints, language skills, low quality scientific publications at the national and regional levels, and poor access to the Internet.

3.7 What else is needed to improve health research systems?

The framework for a health research system introduced in Chapter 1 outlines a set of concepts to help map out key functions and areas for policy-making. The previous sections have elaborated on these functions and suggested various ways they could be developed and strengthened. But in order to improve health research systems, other areas that cut across all four functions also need attention.

Figure 3.9 Bona Simanjuntak gives a Wi-Fi demonstration to students in Jakarta, Indonesia

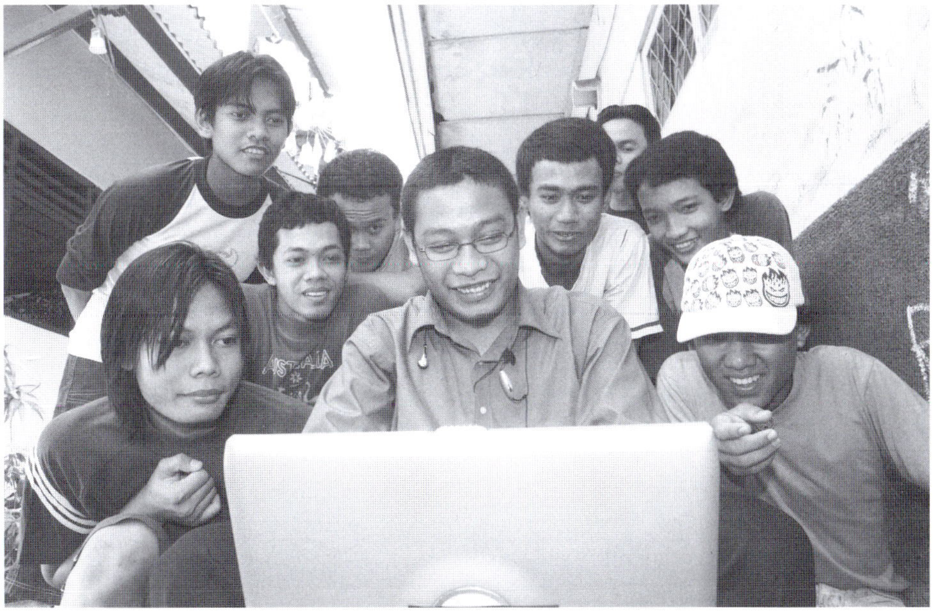

Photo by Edy Purnomo/JiwaFoto.com

Source: Wagstaff J. Wi-Fi is aiming for the masses. *Far Eastern Economic Review*, 2004, June 17, 38-40.

Each country's national health research system varies in terms of the mix of different sectors, organizations, legal and regulatory frameworks, degree of decentralization, social values, historical context, health challenges, among other characteristics and processes. These are all unique to each country. This report proposes that the overall goals of a health research system are to produce and use knowledge for better health. But more specific national goals, policies and strategies are also needed to complement this overarching system goal, taking into account sub-national as well as the regional and international context.

Addressing the need to understand and share experiences on health research systems

Benchmarking of national health research systems may provide one way to complement but not replace qualitative and other contextualized analyses. In general, international and regional benchmarking efforts assume that data and information from a range of countries point toward a new understanding of shared problems; toward new solutions to those problems; or to new mechanisms for implementing policy and improving performance, including cooperation across countries *(15)*. Benchmarks are entry points to interpret and discuss the examples from around the world and often provide invaluable evidence of what works in practice. They can also help avoid either re-inventing the wheel or repeating others' mistakes. Policy- and decision-makers can also learn from the ways in which other governments undertake the process of policy-making itself despite differences in contexts.

Many high-income countries have conducted analyses of selected areas of national health research systems policies and activities, which incorporate benchmarking for the purpose of system improvement. For example, the New Zealand Ministry of Research, Science and Technology commissioned a study to evaluate the appropriateness of the government's strategic investment in the management of health research in order to better inform future policies and strategies *(16)*. The 2004 report notes that there is "no single ideal comparator country" and comparisons are thus made with a range of selected countries: Australia, Canada, Ireland, the Netherlands, Sweden and the United States. Benchmarks, such as levels of financial investment funnelled through medical and health research councils, are discussed in relation to different management and organizational models for the health research system. Based on the analyses conducted, a series of recommendations to further strengthen the existing system are proposed for discussion. These span funding arrangements, performance indicators for health research, and international collaboration, among others.

A better understanding of national health research systems is one means towards recognizing the challenges and developing policies that improve the functioning of a national health research system. Part of this improvement requires that the health research system's various functions operate together to achieve a common set of goals. The reality is that in most countries, especially in low-income and many middle-income countries, data sources and organizational analyses on health research are limited. In such cases, existing reports and reviews do not provide a comprehensive view of health research as an input to strengthen the system. Even less attention is given to how to strengthen the links between the health research system and the health system to produce knowledge for better health.

Drawing on many of the previous experiences cited in this chapter, WHO in close collaboration with interested member states is developing and testing a policy-oriented benchmarking approach for low- and middle income countries (see Box 3.14). This collective benchmarking aims to achieve two goals and is part of a strategy to build national capacity to investigate, discuss and analyse health research activities and policies. The first goal is to develop new ways of gathering good quality comparative information on a selected set of indicators that are relevant to health research goals in low- and middle-income countries. Besides quantitative indicators, this also includes qualitative information and

Box 3.14 Collective benchmarking of health research systems

WHO's health research system analyses (HRSA) team is currently developing methods to analyse the processes involved in the management, production and utilization of health research. This initiative, in collaboration with many partners, also seeks to promote the notion that health research is organized in a system.

As part of the project, the HRSA is conducting a pilot study involving 13 low- and middle-income countries: Brazil, Cameroon, Costa Rica, Indonesia, Iran, Kazakhstan, Laos, Malaysia, Pakistan, the Russian Federation, Senegal, Tanzania, and Thailand (the focal points and national teams involved in this project are listed on the report's web site www.who.int/rpc/wr2004). This group of 13 countries is referred to throughout the chapter, with some preliminary results provided from the pilot study. Although Australia and New Zealand are not among the 13 countries involved in the study, they contributed towards this benchmarking effort.

The pilot phase of this study has two goals. One is to develop a collective benchmarking approach to identify and test basic indicators that describe national health research systems across all participating countries. These indicators include not only quantitative data, but also qualitative information and processes specific to each national context. The second goal is to assemble or strengthen national task forces on health research, which ideally would include representatives with an array of perspectives, from both public and private sectors. Besides stimulating national, regional and international discussions among a broad range of stakeholders on the interpretation and policy relevance of the study for health research systems and health systems, the establishment of the task forces would serve as a means to further institutionalize the monitoring and evaluation of health research systems.

In an effort to establish a benchmarking system, a set of 14 core indicators and 42 descriptive variables were devised in 2002 building on existing approaches to evaluate research investments.* Each of these indicators and variables relates to one of the four main functions of a health research system: 1) stewardship, 2) financing, 3) human and institutional capacity, and 4) producing and utilizing research. For instance, core indicators that are part of the stewardship function include:

- Is there a national policy on health research that integrates the perspectives of all key stakeholders?
- Is there a forum or process to coordinate the setting of national health research priorities?
- Do ethical review boards exist?
- Are there monitoring and evaluation activities clearly linked with strengthening health research systems?

In addition to the collection of existing data, a portfolio of additional approaches to describing and analysing health research systems has been under development as part of the benchmarking initiative. This portfolio includes policy reviews, new approaches to analyse reference databases, media coverage assessments, focus group discussions and assessments of the utilization of health research. Workshops for the national teams to discuss progress on collective benchmarking were due to be held in September and October 2004.

* European Commission 2001. *Indicators for benchmarking of national research policies: key figures 2001.* Unit for Competitiveness, Economic Analysis and Indicators, Research Directorate General, Brussels, Belgium. UNESCO 2002. *Science & technology statistics and indicators in developing countries: perspectives and challenges*, UIS/S&T/2/BD1, UNESCO Institute for Statistics, Montreal, Canada.

processes that are specific to each national context. The second is to further stimulate national, regional and international discussion with a broad range of stakeholders, on the interpretation of information as well as the policy relevance of the process for the health research system and the health system.

The indicators selected for further development and testing also build on the recommendations of the Commission on Health Research for Development. For example, based on the evidence presented in its 1990 Report, the Commission concluded that key areas for strengthening in low- and middle-income countries include the range of health research fields, range of outputs, capacities, quality of research, training, supporting environment, and research dissemination and use *(17)*.

The benchmarking process and involvement of a wide range of stakeholders also recognizes and builds on subsequent activities stimulated by the Council on Health Research for Development and other organizations that have supported extensive discussions of ENHR *(18)* and research capacity building in low- and middle-income countries. For example, many WHO Regional Offices, including the Eastern Mediterranean and South-East Asian regions, have sponsored case studies and policy discussions on health research systems.

The way forward

Benchmarking and broad stakeholder discussions are examples of important tools and processes that could help improve health research systems if used to improve and inform policies. They are a means to an end, rather than an end in themselves. Other examples of what is needed to inform the health research system include:

- analysing the ways in which different parts of the system interact;
- promoting better links with the broader research system and science and technology in general;
- improving interaction with private sector and civil society research;
- creating innovative models of organization, such as networks of centres of excellence;
- reducing corruption by improving transparency and accountability.

But even the best-organized health research system must ultimately use knowledge to deliver improved health outcomes. This is the subject of Chapter 4.

References

1. Paraje G et al. Produccion cientifica en el area OPS (Scientific production in the AMRO Region). Presented at the First Latin American Workshop on Indicators of Science, Technology and Innovation in Health, organized by RICYT and the Pan American Health Organization, Buenos Aires, September 2004. HRSA study group. Individual survey results. 2004
2. WHO Health Research System Analyses team and project group: preliminary results, 2004.
3. Stokes D. *Pasteur's quadrant*. Washington, DC, Brookings Institution Press, 1997.

4. D'Souza C, Sadana R. Overview of case studies on health research systems in low- and middle-income countries. Research Policy and Cooperation background document (in review). Geneva, World Health Organization, 2004.
5. WHO Health Research System Analyses team and project group. Preliminary results. 2004
6. *Monitoring Financial Flows for Health Research*. Geneva, Global Forum for Health Research, 2001.
7. WHO, World Bank, and USAID. Guide to producing national health accounts with special applications for low-income and middle-income countries. Geneva, 2003.
8. Canberra Manual: Manual on the measurement of human resources devoted to Science and Technology. Paris, Organisation for Economic Cooperation and Development [OECD/GD(95)77], 1995.
9. Outward bound. *The Economist*, September 28, 2002.
10. Sadana R et al. Importance of health research in South Asia. *British Medical Journal*, 2004, 328:826–830.
11. Hyder AA et al. Capacity development for health research in Pakistan: the effects of doctoral training. *Health Policy and Planning*, 2003, 18:338–343.
12. WHO Health Research Systems Analyses team and project group: preliminary results, 2004.
13. Haines A et al. Bridging the implementation gap between knowledge and action for health. *Bulletin of the World Health Organization*, 2004, 82:724–732.
14. More information about the Cochrane Health Promotion and Public Health Field may be obtained at: www.vichealth.vic.gov.au/cochrane/about/scope.htm, including the complete list of existing systematic reviews and protocols (reviews in progress) at: www.vichealth.vic.gov.au/cochrane/activities/review.htm
15. Wait S. *Benchmarking: a policy analysis*. London, The Nuffield Trust, 2004.
16. *Science for Life: an evaluation of New Zealand's Health Research Investment System based on International Benchmarks*. Australian Expert Group in Industry Studies, University of Western Sydney, 2004.
17. Commission on Health Research for Development. *Health research: essential link to equity in development*. Cambridge, MA, Oxford University Press, 1990.
18. *ENHR: Essential National Health Research—a strategy for action in health and human development*. Task Force on Health Research for Development Secretariat, Geneva, 1991.

4

Linking Research to Action

"As studies have shown, evidence is rarely applied to decision-making in accordance with a rational linear model. In practice, evidence is often generated through doing—in the enactment of policy. Evidence may be only one component of any decision-making process, but it can be made an integral part of a culture of inquiry based on continual learning and development."
(David Hunter and Amanda Killoran)

"Knowledge is not a commodity—it does not flow down a gradient from researchers to decision-makers. Using a soccer metaphor, management of knowledge is not about keeping an eye on the ball but on the goal, and being sensitive to the nature and vagaries of the playing field. Knowledge is not the ball but what goes on between the players who share a belief and a common purpose—to score the goal."
(Ariel Pablos-Mendez)

Key Messages

- Researchers and research organizations need the skills and resources to communicate with users in a more effective way. Funders could support this by making effective communication of relevant research results mandatory.
- An environment must be created where the users of research can access and find relevant research to inform their decisions. The main users of research are the public, civil society/NGOs, patients, medical staff, health system managers, health insurers, researchers, and policy-makers.

Interesting numbers

264 years	Time taken between James Lancaster's discovery that lemon juice prevented scurvy and the British Navy's decision to ensure an adequate supply of citrus fruits on navy ships.
30–40%	Percentage of patients in the United States and Europe who fail to receive cost-effective interventions justified by the best-available scientific evidence.
Doubled	Number of high-quality studies on complex health system interventions available after a systematic review included a search of the "grey" literature.
25%	Percentage of patients in some Asia-Pacific countries with unstable angina or a previous myocardial infarction taking beta-blockers despite strong evidence for the efficacy of this safe and cheap medication.
2–15%	Percentage of African children sleeping under bednets in 2001.

(Sources for these numbers are given on the report web site: www.who.int/rpc/wr2004)

- The producers and users of health research should work more closely together to shape the research agenda and to ensure that research is used to improve health.
- Intermediaries, or knowledge "brokers", can build and nurture relationships between producers and users of research. The media can also help in this.
- Not enough is known about the effectiveness of health strategies in low-income countries, therefore, more investment is needed to evaluate their impact.
- Communities can be a powerful influence on governments to accept change, particularly in the developing world. Attempting to implement a health improvement programme without community support could result in failure.

4.1 Understanding the links between research, policy, practice and public opinion

The word "research" frequently conjures up images of bespectacled scientists in white overalls toiling in laboratories among test tubes and high-tech equipment. There is usually little appreciation of how knowledge produced from research is actually used or translated to improve health *(1,2,3)*. Just as little is known about whether current ways of promoting research findings are effective, especially in developing countries.

In this respect, knowledge management has become an important strategy to ensuring that knowledge produced by the health research system (Chapter 3) is used to improve health. What does knowledge management mean? Introduced in Section 3.1, this refers not only to the body of knowledge but how this knowledge is systematically collected and archived, disseminated, accessed, synthesized and utilized. In addition to the well-known use of knowledge to develop drugs, vaccines, diagnostics, devices and other interventions, it also includes knowledge utilization to inform policy, practice and public opinion. In particular, it includes the key notion of how to promote knowledge-based change in a health system.

Positive change does not automatically result from sound evidence alone, no matter how well synthesized or how effectively communicated. If it did depend only on this, no one would smoke, or over-eat or drink too much alcohol. Everyone would exercise regularly and always fasten their seat belts. Practitioners would follow guidelines and their patients would comply with prescribed treatment. Governments would ensure that key research findings were widely promoted and used to develop policies and make funding decisions.

The failure to use effective interventions is a global problem *(4,5)*. Studies have shown that up to half of the patients in the United States and Europe are not receiving care according to the best scientific evidence *(6)*. A major study on child survival concluded that around 60% of the 10.8 million deaths among children in 42 low-income countries could be prevented by effective and affordable interventions *(7)*. In 2001, it was estimated that only 2–15% of African children were sleeping under bednets. A separate study in Asia-Pacific countries found that only 25% of patients with unstable angina or a previous myocardial infarction used beta-blockers *(8)*. It also found that the patients who did not use these safe, effective and inexpensive medications were more likely to be in less well-off countries.

The other problem is that the use of ineffective or inefficient treatments may pose significant risk of harm to patients, place additional burdens on over-stretched health services and waste limited resources. The continued use of certain antimalarial drugs despite sound evidence of drug resistance is but one example *(9)*. This is particularly devastating in low-income countries where most people pay for health care out of their own pockets.

The notion of "knowledge for better health", therefore, must go beyond the production and passive dissemination of research. National health research systems should:

- focus more attention on promoting the use of research and on designing research "strategically" to solve priority problems in health
- acknowledge that the users of research also generate knowledge, albeit in different ways, and that they should be closely involved in the research process
- evaluate the different approaches to implementing research findings and interventions in health-care delivery, as well as promoting evidence-based practice. The ultimate goal is the strengthening of health systems *(10)*.

To solve public health problems and change practice, evidence-based recommendations, guidelines and programmes have to be actively and effectively promoted. The pharmaceutical industry has learnt that investment in research and development does not effortlessly lead to successful products. The world's biggest drug makers spend billions of dollars a year on a range of promotional activities based on extensive market research. Market analysis is done in advance and the research process managed accordingly. These activities are, in turn, evaluated on precise outcome and performance measures. In the same way, the findings of scientific research that are not sponsored by a pharmaceutical company have to be communicated and promoted effectively in order to shape public policy, practice and public opinion, and help to solve public-health problems.

While drug companies are successful in marketing and advertising geared towards selling their products, it is questionable, for example, whether they would promote the results of a large trial showing that most people with hypertension should be put on an inexpensive diuretic rather than a costlier treatment. Professional and public education programmes need more funding so that they can spread their important messages with the same success as industry-sponsored marketing campaigns.

Research is essential, but not sufficient, to decide which policies and practices to promote and implement. The links between these two areas are complex and there is no direct route between them (see Figure 4.1). Due to the many factors influencing the process of translating research findings into practice including the actors involved, the social and political environment and financial constraints, no one strategy alone can possibly be effective in all settings.

As noted in Chapter 1, the notion of "knowledge for better health" involves a continuous cycle of research, application and evaluation, and learning from that experience. Where does this learning occur? One of the key contributions of research to health systems is the translation of knowledge into actions: to use research to shape health policies, health practices and public opinion. It is in this environment that such learning and problem-solving can, and should, occur.

Therefore, just as research should inform practice, so too should practice inform research. As Figure 4.2 illustrates, learning opportunities and the

Figure 4.1 Research to policy and practice pathway

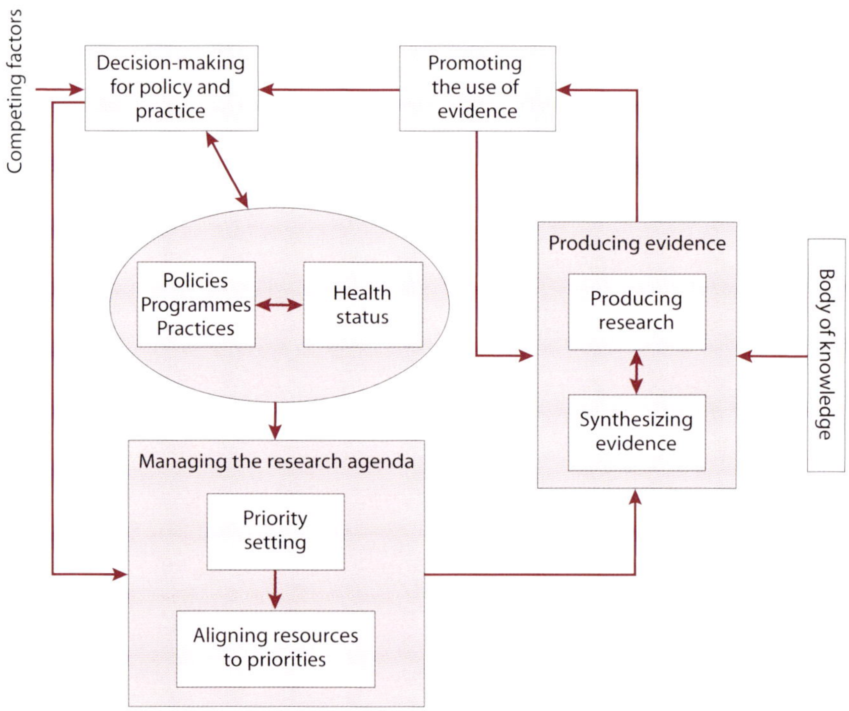

Source: *Strengthening Health Systems: The role and promise of policy and systems research*, Geneva, Alliance for Health Policy and Systems Research, 2004.

experience they bring can significantly influence health outcomes (at least in the clinical setting of hospitals). Operational or field research (in households and communities, in consultations between practitioner and patient, in hospital administration, in the ministry of health and in the international arena), for example, can identify questions and challenges that need to be addressed through future research.

This chapter examines the barriers that may prevent the use of knowledge. It looks at what producers and users of research can do to improve the chances that evidence generated will be acted on. It also highlights the key role research should play in implementing and evaluating policies, programmes and interventions. Much of the research underpinning the approaches described in this chapter, however, was conducted in high-income countries and more research of this kind is needed in low- and middle-income countries.

There is simply not enough evidence to systematically review, reach definitive conclusions or establish what may be the "best practices" in this field. This is reflected in the fact that case studies are often used to highlight links between health research and policy *(11,12)*. In the same vein, several illustrative examples from the developing world have been chosen in the present chapter to show the broad diversity of health research and the beneficial impact research can have when acted on.

Figure 4.2 Experience matters: links between mortality rate and volume of surgical procedures

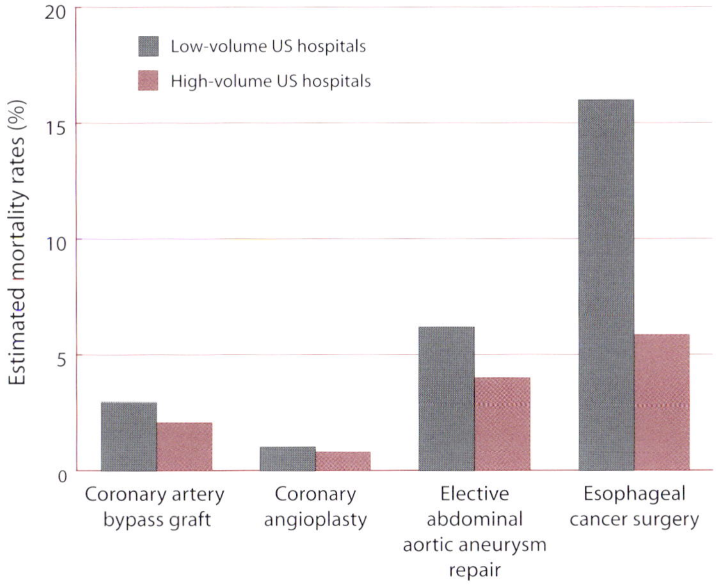

Source: Birkmeyer JD. *Leapfrog patient safety standards: the potential benefits of universal adoption*. Washington, DC, The Leapfrog Group for Patient Safety, 2000.

4.2 Challenges and barriers to the use of research

There are significant challenges associated with bridging the gap between knowledge and action *(1,2,3)*. Decision-making processes are complex. Knowledge, or evidence, is only one contributing factor to how policies are shaped, how health workers practise and how people make decisions concerning their health. Research knowledge must often compete with other factors including beliefs, intuition, habits, superstitions, traditions, past experiences, culture, personal interests and political considerations. Ultimately, however, scientific evidence should help to enlighten and complement the more cultural and personal beliefs and values people hold.

The processes through which knowledge is transferred, taken up and exchanged among individuals and groups are also complex:

- Practitioners, for example, work in many contexts apart from interacting with their patients: they work within a regulatory environment (e.g. pharmacies may be able to dispense medication directly to patients without a prescription), an administrative environment (e.g. a hospital or clinic may set its own rules for how a particular service will be provided), a community environment (e.g. a village or town may rally behind a call for a particular service), and an educational environment (e.g. a practitioner may turn to a respected colleague for advice or seek formal continuing education) *(13)*.
- Public policy-makers also work within a particular institutional structure that makes some options feasible and others virtually impossible. For example, a political system with many checks and balances can make it possible for a single group to mobilize or veto a proposal. Policy-makers also face competing interests from international donors, pharmaceutical companies, NGOs, physicians, patient groups, and civil society groups, and many conflicting ideas about what should be done and why *(14)*.

Table 4.1 illustrates some of the potentially conflicting interests of policy-makers and researchers *(15)*. In Box 4.1, Daniel M. Fox, President of the Milbank Memorial Fund, gives his views on the problem and makes a few

Table 4.1 Conflicting interests of policy-makers and researchers

Policy-makers	*Researchers*
Complex policy problems	Simplification of the problem
Focused solutions	Interest in related but separated issues
Reducing uncertainties	Finding the truth
Speed	Time to think
Control and delay	Publish or perish
Manipulation	Explanation
Feasible and pragmatic solutions	Thoughtful deliberations

Source: Bensing JM. Doing the right thing and doing it right: toward a framework for assessing the policy relevance of health services research. *International Journal of Technology Assessment in Health Care*, 2003, 19:604–612.

Box 4.1 Research to policy: a contrarian's view

Most discussions about doing research that is relevant to policy or communicating research results to policy-makers are self-referential discussions about researchers and their problems. I work with policy-makers who say: "This is what I must decide by this deadline: who can tell me something that may help me make a decision that meets my criteria?" Their criteria often include improving health care and population health, but they always address health status in the context of retaining office or acquiring more resources and authority, or just surviving. Most policy-makers are eager to use the best available information, but someone they trust has to know how and from whom to get that information—and how to present and communicate it.

Many policy-makers readily agree that it would be useful to have research that increases the possibility that information they may want to use will be available in the future. But policy-makers who allocate resources to and within the health sector usually cannot act on this platitude because they have too many pressures on them to act now on other matters.

How, then, can we close the gap between policy-making for health care and population health and researchers? Possibilities include:

- Dramatizing, with anecdotes and examples, problems that would be addressed more effectively if policy-makers allocated resources in advance.
- Funders Forums are helpful if the members include, or have close working relationships with, persons who fund health services and hence know what service funders' priorities are. Be aware, however, that policy-makers need to develop considerable trust before they say what problems are actually bothering them. This is because they do not really believe that researchers will suggest a fresh way to address any of those problems in a timely way.
- Formal knowledge brokerage systems (and professional brokers) are more likely to inform clinical practice and clinical policy within an institution than they are to inform policy-making for health services. Policy-makers do not look around for a broker when they are under pressure to make a decision, which they always are. They look to their staff who either know or do not know how to find and use the best available evidence. Researchers who inform policy have the technical and social skills—and the motivation—to act as temporary, informal advisers to policy-makers and their staff.
- Finally, it is artificial, but frequently it is good politics to separate, as clearly as possible, research on interventions to prevent, diagnose or treat disease from research on health systems and services more broadly. Policy-makers often regard research on prevention, diagnosis and treatment as more separable from politics and commerce than research on systems and services. Moreover, the methodology of primary research and research synthesis on prevention and treatment has reached a level of sophistication at which the word "confidence" can have roughly the same functional meaning to policy-makers and biostatisticians.

Source: Daniel M. Fox, President, Milbank Memorial Fund.

suggestions as to how researchers could more effectively communicate with policy-makers.

Table 4.2 lists other possible barriers to the use of research *(3)*. The relative importance of each of these barriers varies between countries and among users depending on the nature of the research findings and the constraints facing a nation's health system. For example, low- and middle-income countries do not have the financial resources to pay for expensive medicines that have been proven to be effective and that are widely available in high-income countries. Similarly, lack of advanced technology and the shortage of health workers create formidable barriers to implementing research findings in low- and middle-income countries. However, these factors may be less critical for delivering basic interventions such as vaccines.

Some factors that may be perceived as barriers can also act as levers for change. For example, patients may influence practitioners' behaviour towards better practice by requesting interventions of proven effectiveness. Practitioners may be influenced positively when cost-effective interventions are promoted by the media.

Using research in low- and middle-income countries with health systems

Table 4.2 Potential barriers to uptake of evidence by health professionals

Barriers may exist in the:

Health-care system

- Lack of financial resources
- Inappropriate financial incentives
- Inadequate human resources (quantity and quality)
- Lack of access to care
- Health policies that fail to promote cost-effective interventions or advocate unproven activities
- Failure to provide practitioners with access to appropriate information

Practice environment

- Limitations of time
- Poor practice organization, for example there may be a lack of disease registers or mechanisms to monitor repeat prescribing

Educational environment

- Failure of curricula to reflect research evidence
- Inappropriate continuing education and failure to link up with programmes to promote quality of care
- Lack of incentives to participate in effective educational activities
- Influence of commercial interests may bias educational activities

Social environment

- Influence of media may create inappropriate demands/beliefs
- Influence of social fads and trends
- Impact of disadvantage on patients' access to care, literacy and health behaviours

Political environment

- Ideological beliefs may be inconsistent with research evidence
- Political corruption
- Short-term thinking may dominate

Practitioner

- Obsolete knowledge
- Influence of opinion leaders may go against research evidence
- Beliefs and attitudes (for example, these may be related to previous adverse experience of innovation)

Patient

- Demands for ineffective care
- Perceptions or cultural beliefs about appropriate care

Source: Haines A et al. Bridging the implementation gap between knowledge and action for health. *Bulletin of the World Health Organization*, 2004, 82:724–732.

that are chronically under-funded, under-staffed and poorly regulated presents additional challenges. In terms of addressing the most pressing health-care needs of the majority of people in the developing world, the gap between what is known and what remains to be known about effective interventions may be significantly less than the gap between what is known and what is actually being done. Given the huge potential to save the lives of millions of people and improve the health of many more, finding cost-effective ways to promote the use of evidence-based interventions should be a priority for researchers, policy-makers, practitioners and civil society alike *(3)*. Evidence-based practice is particularly important in low-income settings because limited resources must not be wasted *(16)*.

To best meet this challenge, producers and users of research should work more closely together. It is vital for producers of research, including funders and researchers, to take more responsibility for communicating the need to use evidence-based research in a more effective way. In the same way, policy-makers and others who use research need to seek out research that is relevant to their decisions.

4.3 How can researchers effectively communicate research results?

"Knowledge is... a species of money, which is valued greatly, but only adds to our well-being in proportion as it is communicated..."
(Jean-Jacques Rousseau)

Communicate research results in a user-friendly way

The producers of research such as scientists and the institutions where they work can facilitate the use of research knowledge by thinking carefully about what should be transferred, to whom, by whom, how, and with what effect *(17)*. Historically most producers of research have sought to transfer the results of a single study to an undifferentiated group of "decision-makers". Typically they have done this on their own, using "passive" strategies like mailing a copy of a study report without explaining the potential impact of the research, or how they would measure whether their goal had been achieved. But a different approach may be more effective and less likely to do harm. The following five-step approach for more effective transfer of research results has been proposed by Lavis *(17)*: developing a message based on systematic reviews that can be acted upon, identifying the most appropriate target audience, using credible messengers, using proven approaches to transferring the message, and evaluating the impact of that message (see Box 4.2).

Members of the Bellagio Child Survival Study Group and the Multi-Country Evaluation of IMCI Study Group wrote five articles in the *Lancet* in 2003 that looked at how to achieve the MDG of reducing child mortality by two thirds between 1990 and 2015 *(7,18,19,20,21)*. Embedded in the articles was a clear message for public policy-makers and those who seek to influence them. The message can be stated in a four-sentence paragraph that tells a busy public policy-maker the four things he or she needs to know: 1) what is the issue from the perspective of a decision-maker? 2) what does the research evidence reveal? 3) does current decision-making differ from decision-making informed by this research evidence? and 4) who should act and what should be done? The message is as follows:

Box 4.2 A five-step approach to knowledge transfer

Step 1—the "what" of knowledge transfer

Develop an actionable message based on a body of research knowledge that has been systematically reviewed (when possible), and seek to achieve consensus on the message. Crafting an appropriate message takes great care. It should be based on an assessment of the potential benefits of a course of action weighed against the potential harm and costs, and, if possible, should also be based on an assessment of its applicability across groups. The Cochrane Collaboration has begun to develop methods to standardize the assessment and reporting of health equity factors in systematic reviews, including how to assess and report differences in intervention effect across socioeconomic gradients and how to assess and report the effects of interventions targeted at the socioeconomically disadvantaged.

Step 2—"to whom"

Identify the most appropriate target audiences for a message and fine-tune the message and the approach to knowledge transfer for each target audience. The balance between top-down initiatives, that is initiatives focused on public policy-makers and bottom-up initiatives which are initiatives focused on the general public, patients, and health-care providers as a means of bringing about change in health systems will depend on existing capacities as well as interest in the topic.

Step 3—"by whom"

Identify and work with or through the most credible messengers for each combination of message and target audience. Researchers with the skills and inclination to engage in knowledge transfer may be the most credible messenger for some, but likely not all, target audiences. Former public policy-makers who have credibility among both the research community and the current pool of public policy-makers may be the most appropriate messenger for this target audience. The executive director of an NGO may be the most appropriate messenger for other NGOs. Clinical opinion leaders may be good messengers for practitioners and some popular media personalities may be good messengers for the general public. Individuals who have experience in multiple roles, particularly as both researchers and decision-makers, may be particularly well placed to act as credible messengers. But there are no certainties here. Perceived credibility comes from many sources and may need to be determined locally and/or separately for different types of situations.

Step 4—"how"

Almost all of the proven approaches to transferring messages to target audiences involve some type of face-to-face interaction. For knowledge transfer to health-care providers, systematic reviews of randomized controlled trials now exist to assist in the selection of possible interventions. These interventions typically improve care by an order of 10%. That said, the trials have been conducted primarily in high-income countries, the cost-effectiveness of implementing proven approaches in particular contexts has typically not been examined prior to implementation, and scaling-up efforts have not been well documented. For knowledge transfer to health-system managers and public policy-makers, a systematic review of observational studies has reinforced the importance of face-to-face interaction for these two target audiences. But the optimal design of these interactions has yet to be determined. Small-scale qualitative research may help anticipate the key barriers to uptake of specific research findings in a given setting and suggest strategies for overcoming these obstacles.

Step 5—"with what effect"

Articulate the impact that knowledge transfer efforts are trying to achieve, evaluate whether the impact was achieved and share evaluation experiences with others. Changing clinical practice can be seen as an appropriate objective when an intervention is clearly unsafe or ineffective. In other circumstances, informing patient decision-making can be seen as an appropriate objective because patients' values may lead them to choose one intervention offered to them by a clinician over another intervention. Informing political debate, not successfully changing or introducing a public policy, can be seen as an appropriate objective in democracies because societal values, as well as who wins and who loses, matters in public policy-making.

Source: Lavis J et al. How can research organizations more effectively transfer research knowledge to decision makers? *Milbank Quarterly*, 2003, 81:221–248.

- Forty-two countries accounted for 90% of the 10.8 million child deaths in 2000 and most of the deaths could have been prevented if simple, effective and cheap interventions had reached all children who needed them.

- Making 15 preventive interventions and eight treatment interventions universally available in the 42 countries with 90% of child deaths worldwide in 2000 would reduce child mortality by 63% and thereby achieve one of the eight MDGs.

- Global coverage for most interventions is below 50% but universal coverage is achievable.
- Public policy-makers in the 42 countries should consider whether the 15 preventive and eight treatment interventions should be applied to their country context. They should examine the possibility of tailoring delivery strategies for the interventions to their stage of health system development to achieve universal coverage of the interventions, and should consider commissioning additional research when optimal delivery strategies are not known.

Effective communication can speed up the use of research findings in the field. Recommendations based on research results need to be made understandable to potential users. The traditional approach used by researchers is the peer reviewed journal, which involves describing the background, methods, results, and discussion points related to a study before offering the study's implications. This approach holds little practical value for decision-makers who do not usually read scientific journals. Instead, brief summaries should be provided that begin with the implications of the research and provide policy options and choices. Additional details can be provided separately for those who want to know more and for those who want to assess the quality and applicability of the research underpinning the message.

Researchers should learn from the pharmaceutical industry which produces and distributes glossy pamphlets with the key features and advantages of their products, along with reprints of published scientific papers supporting their claims. Practitioners or policy-makers are not likely to read those scientific papers, but are reassured by the perception that the information on the glossy folder is based on a reputable publication.

Two important challenges confront the developers and proponents of messages that can be acted on. Firstly they should consider how best to bundle research into messages for a given health system and how best to phase in the messages when the health system cannot support all of them at one time. Secondly, the developers and proponents of a message should be publicly accountable for the veracity and appropriateness of their claims *(22)*. Just as the peer review process is needed to assess the validity of claims based on a single study, a process that brings together the producers and users of research may be needed to assess the validity of a particular message and its appropriateness for a particular context.

Developing, transferring and making available messages that can be acted on (known as "actionable") would require only a small augmentation or reorientation of research funds. The knowledge pyramid below captures the relative balance that a health research system could seek to achieve.

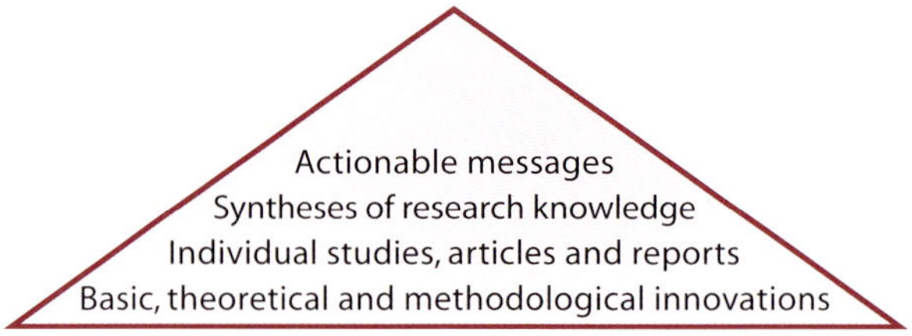

Investments in developing "actionable" messages would be promoted if highly visible organizations required that trial results should always be presented within a Cochrane systematic review that puts the results in perspective, as for example the WHO's Department of Reproductive Health and Research has mandated for the research it funds or produces. Investments in efforts to transfer "actionable" messages could be channeled either through stand-alone funding allocations or, when the probability is high that a single study will yield an "actionable" message (e.g. operations research), through project funding allocations. A small investment in the apex of the knowledge pyramid, however, must be balanced by continued large investments in the base of the knowledge pyramid. The future flow of "actionable" messages depends on both the current stock and future flows of basic, theoretical and methodological innovations, individual studies, articles and reports, and syntheses of research knowledge.

There are several ways to promote the use of research. Selecting the best approach for the topic and the context requires an understanding of why current patterns of policy and practice exist. Moreover, the strategy selected must be consistent with the local context and the behaviour to be targeted. The media, for example, can have a powerful influence on the behaviour of policy-makers, practitioners, industry and the general public. Educational programmes can influence practitioners and the public. In middle- and high-income countries, the European Observatory on Health Systems and Policies has been experimenting with a method known as "rapid reaction evidence seminars", while the Robert Wood Johnson Foundation in the United States has been experimenting with an approach called "safe harbour policy forums." Both approaches bring researchers and policy-makers together to informally discuss a body of research and its implications.

Marketing and advertising are widely used to inform the public of research findings and influence their opinion on health issues. The impact of such advertising on health may be positive or negative depending on the nature of the product. Special events, for example, that bring together researchers, traditional healers, village elders and others have proved to be an effective way of conveying evidence-based health messages to communities. In many of these contexts, an "actionable" message constitutes the starting point for a discussion because only rarely can the originator of the message predict the full range of incentives and constraints faced by decision-makers.

Role of knowledge brokers

Crafting appropriate messages and delivering them to various target audiences is, however, time-consuming and costly, and requires a different set of skills to those needed to conduct research. Most researchers are ill-equipped to do this on their own. This vital task is often best left to professional communicators, intermediaries or "brokers" *(23,24,25)* whose job is to translate and disseminate research findings in an accessible form that can be used by policy-makers and others. Developing countries need to invest more resources to build up these communication skills.

Such efforts can be undertaken with both short-term and long-term objectives. If an "actionable" message is consistent (or at least not inconsistent) with the views of the governing party it can be reasonably expected to inform a political debate. On the other hand, if a message goes against prevailing views, a long-term goal of merely getting the issue on the agenda of the government, an interest group or the general public may be all that can be achieved. Being ready with a message and approach to knowledge transfer in case the government changes or another event changes the political landscape, however, can allow the producers of research to take advantage of windows of opportunity.

4.4 Strengthening the use of evidence in decision-making

The main users of research are the general public, patients, communities, health-care workers, health system and NGO managers, policy-makers and the scientific community. This section focuses primarily on public policy-makers and health system managers. Boxes 4.3 and 4.4 give two examples of how research can inform policy in the areas of health service delivery and noncommunicable disease.

Policy-makers and health system managers can be more effectively supported to use research knowledge in their decision-making in three ways:

- by developing their or their representatives' capacity to use research knowledge;
- by commissioning research or research syntheses when none exist;
- by combining research knowledge with other types of knowledge to bring about change in health systems to achieve health equity.

Firstly, using research requires having the capacity to access the relevant knowledge. For example, in electronic databases such as the Cochrane Collaboration, the NHS Centre for Reviews and Dissemination, the Campbell Collaboration, WHO's Health Evidence Network (HEN), Reproductive Health Library (RHL) and SciELO (Scientific Library Online) in Latin America. Critical appraisal skills and tools are also required to assess the quality of the research or, as is more likely to be the case, to identify high-quality research

Box 4.3 Evidence-based health policy in Mexico

A study conducted in 1999 *(1)* was specifically designed to compare two Mexican institutions providing health care to poor populations: the Ministry of Health (MOH) and the Solidarity branch of the Social Security System (IMSS-OP).

The study's main aim was to determine which was the most cost-effective institution. It was conducted in four states by examining comparable units from each institution. These units served populations with similar characteristics of poverty and the vast majority of users were dependent on free services offered by both systems.

The study found that the availability of resources was better in the system run by the MOH, where there were more health-care workers and hospital beds. The staff in the IMSS-OP system, however, tended to perform better than MOH staff in terms of productivity.

The IMSS-OP system demonstrated higher coverage of basic health-care programmes (e.g. water and sanitation, antenatal care, drug supply, family planning). The IMSS-OP system better maximized its resources: overall costs per capita of the target population were higher in MOH than in IMSS-OP and the MOH tended to have higher administration costs as well as higher curative care costs. The IMSS-OP system also invested more of its resources in preventative services and training staff. The study found that by focusing on supervision of staff, communication, joint data analysis and annual population surveys the IMSS-OP system served its users more efficiently.

Government policy-makers who are considering reforming their health-care structures need access to this kind of information. A detailed analysis of the health care provided and the costs incurred by the two systems is essential for policy-makers to make informed decisions. Such an analysis can be time-consuming and can demand more resources, but significant improvements in health-care systems are often dependent on such evaluations.

IMSS-OP represented the first generation of health reforms in Mexico, which began in 1943. A second generation of reform in the late 1970s focused on primary health care. The 1990s marked the third generation of reforms with the transition to a model increasingly based on evidence *(2)* and favouring systemic changes. The health system was reorganized through the horizontal integration of three basic functions: leadership, financing and provision. Financing was separated from service provision to promote competition and accountability. Health interventions were evaluated for cost-effectiveness and programmes were designed to improve quality of care, while citizens participated in the provision of their own health care. The evidence-based approach is embodied in the National Health Programme 2001–2006 (NHP 2001–2006), which identifies equity, quality and financial protection as major issues to be tackled by the Mexican health system.

Openness to quality health systems research and stability of leadership in the health sector are key elements of Mexican health sector reform, which has resulted in significant improvements in health outcomes (see figure).

Mortality rate from diarrhoeal diseases in children less than 5 years old in Mexico 1978–1993 *(2)*

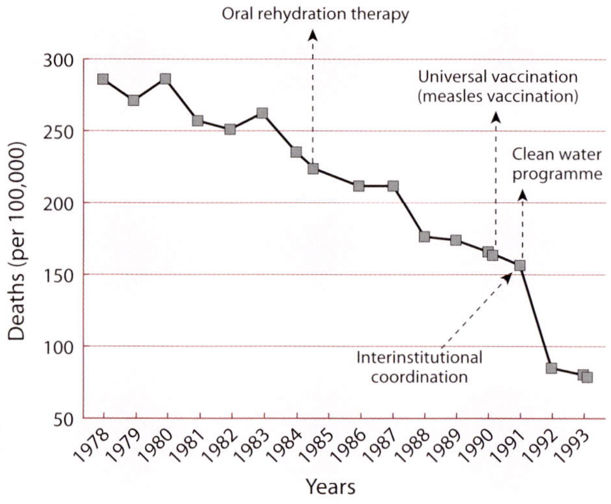

Sources: (1) Kroeger A, Hernandez J M. Health services analysis as a tool for evidence-based policy decisions: the case of the Ministry of Health and Social Security in Mexico. *Tropical Medicine and International Health*, 2003, 8(12):1157–64; (2) Frenk J et al. Evidence-based health policy: three generations of reform in Mexico. *Lancet*, 2003, 362(9396):1667–71.

that has been appraised by others. Often, the research must be adapted to local conditions. For civil servants this adaptation process is typically done when writing briefing notes for politicians.

It is also important to encourage those who make an effort to use research well by ensuring that job descriptions and workplace incentives encourage the use of research. This can also be done by making sure that research plays

Box 4.4 A decade of diabetes research in Cameroon and its political impact

It was not until 10 years ago that the first signs of Cameroon's impending diabetes problem appeared. In 1994, the Health of Population in Transition Research Group (HoPiT)* conducted the country's first epidemiological survey to study the emergence of diabetes and hypertension. Though at the time Cameroon's diabetes prevalence rates were low, the results nevertheless showed that the nation had registered a high enough prevalence of impaired glucose tolerance and diabetes risk factors to warrant concern. Officially, Cameroon was on the verge of a diabetes epidemic. These results spurred much attention, and numerous studies followed, including the Cameroon Burden of Diabetes Project, funded by the World Diabetes Foundation and the NCD (non-communicable disease) Poverty Project, funded by the WHO.

Since then community-based surveys revealed between a 1% to 9% and 0.5% to 0.7% prevalence rate of diabetes in urban and rural areas, respectively (see figure). During an Essential National Health Intervention Project from 1995 to 1999, much evidence was produced for establishing the first diabetes clinics. Staff training guidelines were drafted and tested, as well as follow-up protocols and algorithms. Next, another initiative performed a rapid assessment to improve the detection and management of people with NCDs. In consultation with local health community leaders, this initiative also evaluated patient treatment guidelines in primary health-care centres.

All of these externally funded projects did much to provide valuable baseline information about what was necessary to set up and sustain diabetes clinics. Staff and patient education tools were also created as a result of these projects. In March 2001, Cameroon's Ministry of Health organized a workshop for the dissemination of HoPiT research results to all national health policy leaders. This ultimately resulted in the creation of a department for applied research and a service for NCDs in the disease control department.

There was now adequate political will to label diabetes and hypertension as emerging public health problems, and both were included in the National Ten-Year Health Development Plan. In 2002, a committee was convened specifically to develop a national diabetes policy as well as one for hypertension. After the final consultations for these documents were completed, a workshop was convened in September 2004 to adopt the programmes. While the national diabetes and hypertension policies are to be funded by Cameroon, the World Diabetes Foundation has introduced both a national and regional policy for the surveillance, control and prevention of the disease. Thanks to the efforts of many external partners and donors, in the 10 years since Cameroon's diabetes epidemic was first detected, the country has been able not only to produce the necessary political will to change policy, but to translate research findings into practical health-care programmes.

Prevalence rate of diabetes in urban and rural areas by gender

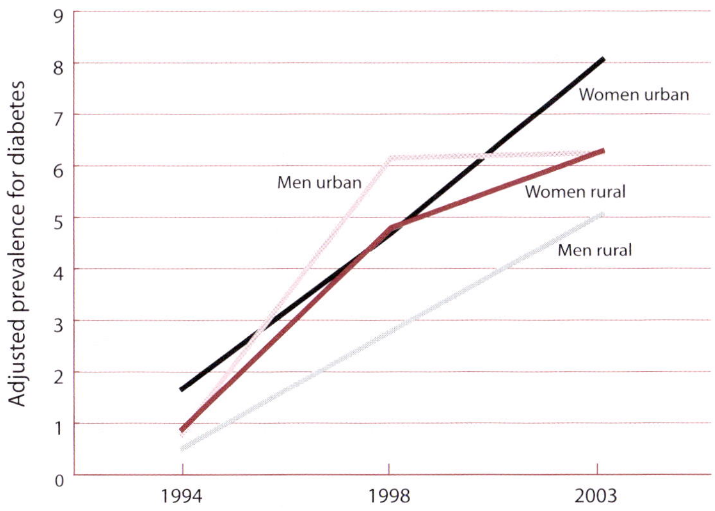

* Health for Populations in Transition (HoPiT) is a research group that was set up to harness the skills and provide evidence-based research for populations in developing and developed countries.

Source: Prof Jean Claude Mbanya, Health of Population in Transition Research Group, Department of International Medicine and Specialities, Faculty of Medicine and Biomedical Sciences, University of Yaoundé I, BP 8046, Yaounde Cameroon. With thanks to Nigel Unwin, Management of Noncommunicable Diseases, WHO, Geneva.

a role in the decision-making process and that sufficient time is allocated to acquire, assess, and adapt research. The Canadian Health Services Research Foundation has developed a self-assessment tool to help organizations evaluate their capacity to use research findings. In a similar move, the Institute for Healthcare Improvement, a US-based champion of evidence-based change, has developed the following seven ways of using research: find sound innovations; find and support "innovators"; invest in "early adopters"; make early adopter activity observable; trust and enable reinvention; create slack for change; and lead by example *(24)*.

Secondly, when gaps are identified in existing information, policy-makers must be supported by the health research system to fill the gaps. This can be done, for example, by commissioning research studies or syntheses. Some examples of areas where more knowledge is needed include development of drugs for neglected diseases and how to better integrate programmes focused on a single disease with the broader health system (see Chapter 2). Another area where gaps might exist is policy-making outside the health sector when there is limited information about social determinants of health, like poverty.

Thirdly, knowledge in several areas must be combined to bring about change in health systems. More specifically, the types of knowledge needed are as follows:

- knowledge about priority problems (e.g. most burdensome diseases);
- knowledge about proven solutions for priority problems (e.g. cost-effective prevention and treatment options for a particular disease profile in a country);
- knowledge about the context for change and whether solutions are likely to work in the local setting (e.g. local interpretation of problems and local capacity to employ particular solutions, where capacity includes human resources, infrastructure, and money);
- knowledge about proven mechanisms to bring about change (e.g. including incentives and building support among the health workforce).

Some users of research may have difficulty in assessing the value of the research about these issues. Politicians, for example, tend to be influenced in their decision-making by how many calls and letters they receive from their constituents and how much media attention an issue is receiving. They tend to evaluate solutions based on what they think is possible in their local context, their own past experiences, the experiences of others, and whether it will improve their chances of re-election.

Two additional points warrant mention. Firstly, the phrase "global evidence for local decisions" needs further clarification. Global evidence about priority problems, solutions, and mechanisms can help bring about change. In contrast, local decisions informed by local knowledge are necessary to create the context for change. The caveat to this phrase is that the applicability of global evidence needs to be assessed for each local context and operations research is needed when the research cannot be applied locally. Joseph Stiglitz captured this well with the title for his keynote address at the first Global Development Network conference: "Scan globally, reinvent locally: knowledge infrastructure and the localization of knowledge."

Secondly, as one moves from individual decision-making to management and public policy-making, knowledge about "the way things are" increasingly competes with values about "the way things should be", and also with private interests. Civil society groups, NGOs, and other groups can identify opportunities for change at the intersection of these competing factors. Over the longer term, they can pressure health system managers and public policy-makers to be accountable to research and to use it as one input in decision-making, in much the same way that health-care providers do. The principles of ethical care require practitioners to make informed decisions or to help their patients make informed decisions. If information about the optimal course of action is lacking, they are supposed to evaluate the outcomes of their chosen course of action. For reasons that are quite legitimate in complex organizations and in governments, managers and public policy-makers could choose courses of action other than those suggested by research. Social pressure, however, could force them to at least make clear the rationale behind the decision and to consider building evaluations into plans to pursue previously unstudied courses of action.

But even the most well-intentioned policy-maker may find it difficult to form evidence-informed health policy because crucial evidence is lacking. Extensive research may be available on the effectiveness of a particular health-care intervention under consideration, but it is a rare occasion when this is matched with evidence on other issues that are important for policy-makers to consider, such as their cost effectiveness, feasibility to implement, cultural appropriateness and effects on health inequalities *(3)*.

Practitioners, patients and the public

Many of the methods outlined above are also relevant for other users of research besides policy-makers. Over the past decade or so researchers in North America and Europe have been working on developing more effective methods to promote professional behaviour change *(25,26)*. For knowledge transfer to health practitioners, systematic reviews of randomized controlled trials now exist to assist in the selection of possible interventions. What has been found is that many of the commonly used approaches to keeping practitioners informed have minimal or unpredictable effects. For example, mailing guidelines or other reports to practitioners has only a small effect on clinical practice, while traditional educational approaches, such as short courses or conferences, have mixed results *(3)*. For its part, the drug industry uses medical representatives and key opinion leaders to deliver messages to health professionals. Research indicates that similarly active dissemination strategies are required if guidelines are to be useful in practice *(3)*. In the developing world, groups like the International Clinical Epidemiology Network (INCLEN) are actively working in this area (see Box 4.5) but to date almost all the trials have been conducted in high-income countries.

What motivates practitioners in wealthy countries to change their behaviour is likely to be very different from what motivates their colleagues in

Box 4.5 INCLEN's Knowledge Plus Project

The Knowledge Plus Program (KPP) of the International Clinical Epidemiology Network, known as INCLEN Trust, promotes better patient care by managing the knowledge base on health interventions using measures of safety, efficacy, effectiveness, efficiency and—equally important—equity and local appropriateness. KPP aims to develop and implement research-driven clinical practice guidelines called Knowledge Plus packages.

The main steps towards the production and use of these guidelines are:

- identification of priority health problems for a specific country and/or region;
- collection of relevant, available literature and information on interventions for these priority problems;
- appraisal of information on such health interventions against benchmarks for efficacy, effectiveness, efficiency, local appropriateness and equity;
- consensus-building among stakeholders on health practice guidelines based on informed appraisal;
- development, dissemination and implementation of Knowledge Plus packages for priority problems;
- monitoring and evaluation.

The "Plus" component of the Knowledge Plus Programme consists of improved tools for assessing local appropriateness and equity, including the use of tacit knowledge. The table shows an example of the appraisal tool used to evaluate equity issues during the examination of the evidence and in the ensuing processes of consensus building, dissemination and feedback.

Knowledge Plus packages are being developed in Colombia, India and the Philippines for acute respiratory infections in children under five years of age, diagnosis of paediatric tuberculosis, management of multidrug-resistant tuberculosis, antiretroviral therapy for HIV/AIDS and management of hypercholesterolemia. These topics were selected because they met the following criteria:

- high probability of successful implementation of practice guidelines in terms of programme feasibility and stakeholder involvement;
- differences in policy and practice among countries in terms of equity and applicability;
- significant equity issues;
- within the interest and expertise of INCLEN members and sufficient evidence available to draft appropriate guidelines.

For more information visit:

www.inclentrust.org/pdf/inclennews/January%202003/INCLEN%20launches%20Knowledge.pdf

www.inclen.org

Applying the KPP equity lens

1. Is the health problem a priority for all stakeholders, including potentially disadvantaged* populations?
2. Did the guidelines look into the possibility of differential effects of treatment (benefits and harms) in potentially disadvantaged populations?
3. Is the voice/interest of potentially disadvantaged populations represented in the expert panel?
4. Is the voice/interest of potentially disadvantaged populations represented in the feedback process?
5. Were feasible knowledge transfer strategies laid out to address barriers to the implementation of the guidelines in potentially disadvantaged populations?
6. Does the impact assessment include evaluation of health gains across potentially disadvantaged populations?

* "Potentially disadvantaged" refers to situations where there may be unfair and avoidable differences in health across populations defined by *any* of the following: (a) Place of residence (e.g., rural, urban, inner-city); (b) Race/ethnicity/culture; (c) Occupation; (d) Gender; (e) Religion; (f) Educational Level; (g) Socioeconomic Status; or (h) Social Capital (e.g., availability of neighborhood support, social stigma, civic society) [Evans T, Brown H. PROGRESS measures of equity, personal communication]

low-income countries. The former are more likely to work in an environment relatively free of economic, personnel or technical constraints while the latter must cope with extremely limited resources, few well-trained personnel and little technology. Nevertheless, with adequate resources, many of the interventions outlined in Box 4.6 could also be applied in developing countries to encourage the use of research by health workers.

The importance of local research can never be underestimated. A survey of physicians in secondary and tertiary hospitals in China, Egypt, Kenya, India and Thailand revealed that local research and publications were most likely to bring about change in clinical practice, followed by North American, European and regional publications *(27)*.

Even less is known about how to assist patients and the public in middle- and low-income countries to use evidence to inform their health-care decisions.

Box 4.6 Translating research findings into practice

- **Educational materials**—Distribution of published or printed recommendations for clinical care, including clinical practice guidelines, audio-visual materials and electronic publications. The materials may have been delivered personally or through personal or mass mailings.
- **Conferences**—Participation of health-care providers in conferences, lectures, workshops or traineeships.
- **Local consensus process**—Inclusion of participating providers in discussions to ensure that they agree that the chosen clinical problem is important and the approach to managing the problem (i.e. the clinical practice guideline or definition of adequate care) is appropriate. The consensus process might also address the design of an intervention to improve performance.
- **Educational outreach visits**—Use of a trained person who meets with providers in their practice settings to provide information with the intent of changing the provider's performance. The information given may include feedback on the provider's performance.
- **Local opinion leaders**—Use of providers nominated by their colleagues as "educationally influential". The investigators must explicitly state that "the opinion leaders were identified by their colleagues".
- **Patient-mediated interventions**—Any intervention aimed at changing the performance of health-care providers where specific information was sought from or given to patients, for example direct mailings to patients; patient counselling delivered by someone other than the targeted providers; clinical information collected from patients by others and given to the provider; educational materials given to patients or placed in waiting rooms.
- **Audit and feedback**—Any summary of clinical performance over a specified period of time. Summarized information may include the average number of diagnostic tests ordered, the average cost per test or per patient, the average number of prescriptions written, the proportion of times a desired clinical action was taken, etc. The summary may also include recommendations for clinical care. The information may be given in a written or verbal format.
- **Reminders (manual or computerized)**—Any intervention that prompts the health-care provider to perform a specific clinical action.
- **Marketing**—Use of personal interviewing, group discussion ("focus groups"), or a survey of targeted providers to identify barriers to change and the subsequent design of an intervention that addresses these barriers.
- **Multifaceted interventions**—Any intervention that includes two or more of the above

Source: Haines A, Donald A, eds. *Getting research findings into practice.* London, BMJ Books, 2nd edition, 2002.

What are their health information needs? What are their priority health issues? The recently formed Global Equity Gauge Alliance is one group attempting to address this gap. It is convinced that community voices must be heard and become part of any strategy to move research to action to improve health and reduce health inequities (see Box 4.7).

4.5 Bringing together the producers and users of research

The existence of structural barriers to effective communication between researchers and decision-makers has been stated previously *(28,29,30,31,32)*. This is a two-way street. Much attention has therefore been focused recently on the idea of creating a more "research-attuned" culture among the users of research and a more "decision-relevant" culture among producers of research by investing in long-term knowledge exchange relationships. Knowledge exchange models have two primary goals: to promote collaborative research and agenda setting, and to promote the application of research to policy and practice. The idea is that the way to close the gap between evidence and clinical practice is by working in partnerships with consumers, health professionals, organizations, researchers and policy-makers. Facilitating interactions between these various groups should increase the use of research findings and lead to research

Box 4.7 Case study: the Equity Gauge Three Pillar Model

In 2002, representatives from 13 countries came together to form the Global Equity Gauge Alliance, an organization committed to reducing health inequities.

The alliance was forged on several convictions:

- that monitoring and continuous advocacy are necessary to raise public consciousness about health inequities;
- that research planning should encompass a strategy for moving research to action with researchers concerned about the use of their work beyond its production and publication;
- that both bottom-up and top-down processes are critical for change;
- that communities have a right to be part of the process of defining priority issues and solutions.

The Equity Gauge's framework to link research to action involves work in three areas:

1. Assessment and monitoring includes identifying priority populations; monitoring progress in reducing inequities over time; and research on interventions and their impact on health inequities
2. Advocacy to highlight health equity issues with decision-makers
3. Support for community empowerment, to ensure that community voices are heard and become part of the solution.

It is when these three areas are integrated that the potential for change is highest (see figure). Regardless of whether an Equity Gauge team is working at a very local level attempting to secure health rights for a population of 10,000 in rural Ecuador, or at an international level seeking solutions to the exodus of doctors and nurses from Africa and Asia, its research to action framework has been shown to be effective.

Developing strong community support for health equity issues in Zambia has helped build political interest and responsiveness. Initially, the Equity Gauge focused on providing technical support to national-level decision-makers, but the team soon realized that without strong public support they would have difficulty in generating a response. And so they began to work on empowering communities by holding a series of meetings to build trust and rapport as well as a level of knowledge about the health-care system and the meaning of health equity.

The Global Equity Gauge Alliance's three-pillar model

The long-term commitment required to achieve results is just one of several lessons that have been learnt in the past two years. At the meeting points of science and politics, academia and civil society, and research dissemination and advocacy tensions are inevitable. Empowering communities to challenge the policy environment while working with government to support pro-poor policy-making requires careful and thoughtful balancing. Sustaining all three pillars has at times been difficult with work seeming to progress more easily in one or two of the pillars, and falling behind in another.

The partnerships that necessarily underpin this broad-based approach can be complex to nurture. In Cape Town, for example, good relationships with the local press resulted in several prominent newspaper articles highlighting the need for redistribution of health resources from privileged to under-resourced areas. But such widespread attention to a sensitive political issue runs the risk of straining working relations with government officials. A large amount of time has to be invested in maintaining trust and avoiding misunderstandings and miscommunication.

For more information, visit www.gega.org.za

Contributed by: David McCoy, Global Equity Gauge Alliance, Durban, South Africa.

agendas that more accurately reflect the priorities of the users of research.

These relationships can involve assuming shared responsibility for setting research priorities and participating in the research process from idea generation through data interpretation. It may also involve participating in the transfer and facilitation of the use of research knowledge, and in formulating, implementing and evaluating the impact of policies. The relationships can also involve the development of a greater awareness of the incentives and constraints operating in each other's worlds, the development of mutual respect for the knowledge that different people bring to the table, and the develop-

Box 4.8 Research to policy: views from senior policy-makers

Evidence and information that could help health policy-makers make decisions is often not readily available when it is needed. One way of addressing the problem is to identify priority areas. Senior health policy-makers, including two ministers of health, met in Kuala Lumpur* in 2004 to discuss information priorities in low- and middle-income countries. The meeting allowed participants to share their experiences in making policy, and, in particular, to discuss how they acquire reliable information and apply it. It also sought ways to promote cooperation between countries in the acquisition and analysis of information. Policy-makers were given two questions to discuss:

1. What were the most important health policy decisions in your country over the past five years? What information could have helped to inform those decisions?
2. What are the most important health policy decisions to be made in your country over the next five years? What information would help to inform those decisions?

The meeting underscored the need shared by all participants for reliable information that could shape policy decisions which could help their countries achieve the MDGs. Participants concluded that:

1. Policy-making is not just about access to the right information or evidence. It can be informed by evidence but it must also take into account other factors which are specific to each country, such as local politics, cultural barriers and the structure and capacity of the health system.
2. Priorities for evidence from the perspective of policy-makers include both health system design issues (e.g., financing, structuring), as well as disease and health issues (e.g., malaria control, infant mortality). Applying best practices and systematic reviews to the specific situation in a given country could improve its use of evidence.
3. More research should be commissioned into health systems in middle- and low-income countries to bridge the gaps in relevant information and evidence. Of critical importance is the allocation of more resources to strengthen capacity to gather and analyze data within ministries of health and other public agencies in those countries. Policy-makers need to be more involved in the design and oversight of that research.
4. WHO should coordinate an international initiative to improve access to and the use of relevant information and evidence to inform health policy decision-making. This should be accomplished through working in partnership with WHO regional and country offices, along with other organizations. More work needs to be done on the national and regional level to create solutions to develop evidence-informed policies.

*Kuala Lumpur, Malaysia, September 16–17, 2004. Senior health policy-makers from the following countries participated: Brunei, China, Georgia, Kenya, Laos, Malaysia, Nigeria, Sudan and Thailand. Co-hosted by the World Health Organization, Milbank Memorial Fund, Centre for Evidence-Based Policy, and the Ministry of Health, Malaysia.

ment of jointly "owned" knowledge about how to improve health systems and achieve health equity.

A recent attempt to assess the information needs of senior health policy-makers from low- and middle-income countries offered some important insights into the key issues (see Box 4.8)

Recent research has also highlighted the importance of ensuring a balance and dialogue between a "data-driven" approach and an "interpretive-translational" approach in which values and assumptions are made explicit and openly debated. This will help to ensure the involvement of the potential users of the research and to assess whether the producers and users of research found the process to be fair and could live with the outcome of the process *(33,28)*.

The main disadvantage associated with the producer and user efforts outlined in sections 4.3 and 4.4 is that they can only go so far because only one "side", the user side, is learning.

Long-term relationships involving the producers and users of research should enhance the relevance and applicability of any research produced and increase the chance that research will be acted upon *(32)*. Proponents of "participatory action research"—a research methodology built around knowledge exchange relationships—have made this point for a long time.

Other research traditions have only recently discovered the point. That said, knowledge exchange is the new "frontier" of bringing research to policy and practice, and this new approach warrants more attention. More evaluation is also needed of innovative practices, such as research funding incentives to foster knowledge exchange relationships, fellowships to encourage researchers to enter policy-making, and "trading places" between researchers and policy-makers for a working day.

Many people are attracted to the knowledge exchange model as the most promising way to bridge the gaps between knowledge (research findings) and action (the reality of policy and clinical practice), and closing large gaps between the care people should receive and the care they do receive. But it really depends on the situation. Sometimes a group effort is not practical or feasible; sometimes a group effort is undesirable. When research conflicts with the dominant point of view, the producers of research may need to go it alone. Getting an issue on the agenda in a hostile environment may be made easier by having a research programme that is independent of the potential users of that research. Either way, the producers of research will still need to develop messages that can be acted upon and undertake many of the other elements associated with communicating the results of research. Similarly, the users of research will still need to develop the capacity to use research knowledge in their decision-making. Confidentiality constraints will often mean that public policy-makers, for example, cannot share freely with researchers the issues they are grappling with. So these are not mutually exclusive options and ideally they should all be pursued.

Observatories, which act as a convenor, middleman or "broker", are one way to bring together the producers and users of research (see Box 4.9). These intermediaries can build and nurture relationships among individuals both within and among organizations with different types of knowledge. Another model called the Reforming States Group (RSG) was convened in 1992 and is a voluntary association of leaders in health policy in the legislative and executive branches of government from most of the states in the USA. The Group aims to share experiences and work on practical solutions to pressing health-care problems *(34)*. Other initiatives in the past, such as the International Health Policy Programme, focused on "pairing" young researchers with policy-makers in the developing world in order to strengthen linkages and better shape health policy *(35)*.

Attributes of personal preparedness, institutional support, and the general climate for knowledge transfer and exchange vary widely in both developed and developing countries *(23)*. Some researchers may be better able to communicate research effectively to non-researchers. Some institutions may encourage scientists to engage in such efforts more than others. Some jurisdictions may be more supportive, such as when the potential users of research consult with researchers when they set research priorities and where resources are specifically allocated for communicating research. Over the long term, civil society

Box 4.9 European Observatory on Health Systems and Policies

Founded in 1998 by WHO's Regional Office for Europe in Copenhagen and other partners including European governmental representatives, the World Bank and the London School of Economics, the European Observatory on Health Care Systems and Policies (based in Brussels, Belgium) draws together available data on public health in order to improve health-care systems in Europe. By contributing to the evolving policy debate on the future of European health-care systems, the Observatory hopes to guide the reform process underway across the continent.

The recognition that country experiences are fundamental to the successful development of public health systems has created new fora for multilateral cooperation between national authorities and international experts. In this way, governments faced with proposed policy changes within their public health structures have rapid access to evidence-based recommendations on the measures taken by other countries facing similar challenges.

The Observatory focuses on three main inter-related areas of work: country monitoring and information, analysis of health system and policy issues, and engagement with policy-makers. To bridge the gap between academic analysis and the practicalities of decision-making, the Observatory seeks to unify methods of data collection as well as to provide common clinical terminology for all practitioners. Such tools are then used by policy-makers to assess the performance of European health-care institutions and make informed decisions about proposed reforms to the public health system.

The Observatory also produces profiles of health-care systems in transition as part of its information and monitoring strategy. These profiles describe and analyse a country's health-care system, that is its organization and funding to facilitate international comparisons. Such profiles bring together researchers and practitioners to analyse major health care issues on a multi-disciplinary basis in order to develop policy recommendations to assist national officials.

Working directly with policy-makers has long been a priority for the Observatory. For instance, for one week in August until 2002 the Observatory ran a specialized "Summer School" in Dubrovnik, Croatia. The programme targeted leading European figures in public health, bringing together representatives from governments, international organizations, and health-care providers, among others. This has since evolved into a series of focused policy dialogues and workshops that provide a unique opportunity for the Observatory to respond to and learn from front-line practitioners. In turn, this practical exchange of information helps to inform countries' decision-making at the policy level.

For more information visit: www.euro.who.int/observatory/Home

groups, NGOs, and other groups can work towards establishing a public accountability for research to be more effectively communicated.

This section and the two preceding sections have focused on the roles of the producers and users of research as well as knowledge brokers in bridging the gaps between research and action, facilitating learning among all players and improving the bi-directional flow of knowledge. The fourth main category of actors—the funders of research—warrants at least a brief mention. Funders of research can create capacity, appropriate incentives, and accountability for researchers with the skills and inclination to engage more effectively in communication efforts. Funders can also create capacity for decision-makers to engage in seeking out research results and participating in the research process, for instance playing a role in setting research questions. And, where possible, funders can create capacity and appropriate incentives for the producers and users of research to engage in knowledge exchange efforts. A knowledge loop connects these four groups of actors and ideally all of them would act together.

In addition, the general public and civil society groups have a role to play beyond their role as users of research. They can exert pressure on the funders and producers of research, on knowledge brokers, and on other users of research (most notably clinicians, health system managers, and public policy-makers) to make sure the knowledge gaps are bridged in the domains most important to them and in ways acceptable to them.

Regional perspective 6

A strong emphasis should be given to improving the linkages between researchers and policy-makers, including the need for developing a cadre of knowledge "brokers" and intermediaries to support national decision-making.

4.6 Improving public health programmes in developing countries

In some cases research is used to make relatively straightforward recommendations. For example:

- policy-makers use research to decide whether a drug or procedure should be included on a national reimbursement list;
- professional societies use research to produce treatment guidelines for practitioners on a particular disease;
- patient advocacy groups use research to educate families about a rare childhood illness;
- health authorities use research to issue a safety warning about a popular over-the-counter herbal treatment.

As discussed in the previous three sections, processes can be enhanced to increase the likelihood that these recommendations will be informed by evidence and effectively communicated to target audiences.

In other cases, research findings are used to develop much broader public health strategies and programmes, which can be far more complex and difficult to implement. For example, a targeted programme aimed at preventing mother-to-child transmission of HIV (PMTCT) involves a number of elements: drugs must be available, health services accessible and used, quality maternal and child health care provided, and adequate HIV testing and counselling services put in place *(3)*. Importantly, such single-disease programmes should not create a maldistribution, or an imbalance, in resources and workforce to the detriment of intended recipients. This is especially a problem in resource-poor countries and Box 1.1 in Chapter 1 gives an example where infants successfully treated with the full PMTCT package subsequently died of congenital syphilis.

In many instances, the distance between taking a policy decision and the improvement in the population's health can be enormous. The implementation of new interventions on a general population basis to control or prevent public health problems raises additional questions and requires further knowledge of health seeking behaviours and cultural and personal beliefs. Using research to reform national health systems to more effectively and equitably deliver and finance health care is equally complex and difficult.

Scaling up special programmes requires a tremendous amount of learning and knowledge generation. Ideally, learning from the field is combined with formal research processes. Complex social systems present research with qualitatively different subjects than is typical in medical science. Traditional research tools such as tightly controlled experiments, randomized double blind trials and standardized interventions are appropriate and effective for investigating a new drug for instance, but these are often difficult to use in the examination of large diffuse social systems such as communities, hospitals and ministries of health. It is not always obvious how to conduct research that would lead to public health improvements and better, more innovative methodologies need to be developed in future (see Section 2.4 for more details)

The way to learn about a system and its operation is by using all available evidence, including evidence generated by the participants in an investigation through an iterative process (a process that repeatedly makes changes and measures their effects over time). This approach to quality improvement is more fluid, more dynamic, less controlled, and less precise than "traditional" research methodology, but it remains fundamentally empirical and is often the only cost-effective and time-effective option.

In fact, operational or field research is being carried out on a continual basis in communities and villages all over the world. Boxes 4.10 and 4.11 illustrate the valuable knowledge that can be gained from the field.

Unfortunately such knowledge is often not documented or shared. Local and international NGOs, donors and lenders collect a wealth of information but much of this research is lost or never known. This is because it is either not published in any form or published in the "grey" literature which is not easily accessible. Grey literature covers a range of published and unpublished material that is not normally identifiable through conventional methods of bibliographic control. A recent study into the cost-effectiveness of routine immunization in low- and middle-income countries showed that the amount of evidence almost doubled after a systematic review of the grey literature. In particular, the evidence was for more complex health system interventions and cost or cost-effectiveness analyses. Interventions described in the grey literature tend to be more up to date, cover a different geographic spread and be published in languages other than English *(36)*.

Processes are needed to systematically collect this knowledge, analyse, summarize and organize it, and then share the information with others. These groups have information as to what happens once a project is implemented and why these programmes often fail to deliver to those in need. A network is needed to make information emerging from operational research available to a wider community quickly, which should help speed up the rate at which new practices or technologies are adopted.

Evaluating the impact of research

As noted by Haines et al. *(3)* there is a lack of evidence on effective implementation strategies in low- and middle-income countries. More investment is thus needed for evaluating such strategies and developing frameworks to evaluate and measure the impact of research, especially health policy, health services and health systems research. This research is just as essential as biomedical research for improving health outcomes.

Evaluating research projects can identify what works and what does not,

Box 4.10 Improving care during pregnancy and delivery

Thailand implements WHO's new model for antenatal care

Antenatal care has long been essential to safeguarding the health of pregnant women and the unborn child. Yet while the standard WHO model of maintaining this has in the past recommended an average of 12 to 16 visits to a health-care provider throughout the course of their pregnancy, a randomized clinical trial surprisingly found that the same level of care is also possible with only four visits.

The WHO systematic review showed that for women without previous or current complications, a sharp reduction in the number of visits is not associated with an increased risk either for woman or child.

This new model of antenatal care would clearly benefit both developed and developing countries, as long as provisions are also made for pregnant women who experience complications or are in emergency situations.

Since the completion of WHO's antenatal randomized care trial, the manual for the implementation of the new model has been published and distributed worldwide. In 2004, Thailand became the first country to adopt this new model of antenatal care following approval from the Royal Thai College of Obstetricians and Gynaecologists and it is currently being implemented, starting with Khon Kaen province.

Source: Villar J et al. WHO antenatal care randomized trial for the evaluation of a new model of routine antenatal care, *Lancet*, 2001, 357:1551–64.

The Better Births Initiative

The Better Births Initiative seeks to implement change in obstetric practice by gaining commitment from policy-makers as well as managers, doctors and midwives working in hospital maternity units. This involves discussions with public health officials and health workers on international trends in evidence-based approaches, sources of evidence, how practice can be improved and the potential impact of change.

The rationale for the Better Births Initiative (BBI) is that if providers change their current practice in relation to a few common obstetric procedures, care would become more evidence-based. These changes could happen today at no cost, and would improve service quality, obstetric outcomes, and women's experience of childbirth.

BBI is a project that started in 2000 in Coronation Hospital in South Africa. Under the initiative, hospital staff in maternity wards considered the potential benefit or harm of procedures used during childbirth and were given a set of evidence-based changes that were achievable with existing resources. The package was presented as an interactive workshop with colourful materials including a workbook, reference booklet, posters, a presentation, video material and a self-assessment mechanism.

A baseline study of current practice helped identify gaps between evidence and practice and areas where change was most needed. Respected peer leaders from individual maternity units were chosen and involved in disseminating agreed changes and institutionalizing new practices. Hospital staff were encouraged to develop mechanisms to ensure quality and monitor progress.

The BBI has undertaken several landmark studies.

In Zimbabwe, a study conducted at a government hospital in Harare used indicators of good obstetric care to help the maternity staff identify gaps between knowledge and actual practice. The study also helped staff identify barriers to implementing research findings at the organizational, social and individual level.

The African Midwives Research Network in Dar Es Salaam, Tanzania, meanwhile, has designed a study to promote the use of more upright positions for birth and mobility during labour. Their study builds on findings from South Africa and will use adapted BBI materials in a training programme to enhance the skills and confidence of midwives to induce them to change their practice.

In China, researchers at the Fudan School of Public Health showed wide variations in clinical practice at government hospitals in Shanghai. Using selected childbirth care procedures in four hospitals, a study compared actual practice against best-practice guidelines and explored user and provider views about each procedure. The study's findings: Obstetric practice is not following best available evidence and there is a need to adjust hospital policy to support the use of interventions of proven benefit to women during childbirth as well as develop approaches that ensure clinical practice changes.

As a result of the study, a process has now been established to try to make obstetric care more evidence-based and arguably, more humane. The Women's Health Care Association of China has conducted an operational study on protecting, promoting and supporting normal birth to encourage evidence-based obstetric care in 13 hospitals nationally. The BBI materials will be translated and adapted for use as a training course in evidence-based childbirth care.

Source: www.liv.ac.uk/lstm/ehcap/BBI/bbimainpage.htm

and why. Armed with this information, necessary adjustments can be made to programme design and when necessary further research can be commissioned. Ideally, evaluation involves a back and forth process of shared experiences, constantly making adjustments and fine-tuning the programme based on the evidence generated and lessons learned. This should first be done on a small scale before it is more widely implemented. Sometimes this process will identify new needs which can then be fed back into the knowledge cycle in the form of a question requiring an evidence-based answer. A recent multi-country evaluation of a major programme (WHO's Integrated Management of Childhood Illness) provided some valuable lessons as to how such evaluations of key public health interventions can be done in the future *(37)*.

How an intervention or programme is evaluated will depend on the health problem being addressed and on the socio-political context, therefore, evalu-

Box 4.11 Field research influences health policy

Since Ghana's Navrongo Health Research Centre (NHRC) participated in the seminal African study on vitamin A supplementation in 1988 it has grown into a world-renowned multi-disciplinary research institution.

In 1992, the Ghanaian Ministry of Health (MOH) adopted the facility with the mandate to investigate population and health problems of both national and international significance, provide advice to policy-makers, and train health personnel.

One of the Centre's ongoing projects, the Community Health and Family Planning Project (CHFP), has significantly contributed to reduced fertility and child mortality rates and consequently facilitated change in the country's national health policy.

In an effort to establish feasible community health service strategies towards achieving Health for All in rural traditional settings in Africa, CHFP was designed to test two sets of under-used resources in sub-Saharan Africa—traditional village-based authority structures and trained health providers in fixed-location clinics—through a four-celled trial in Navrongo, Ghana.

The study area was divided into four districts which were selected to ensure that each cell began the field trial with equivalent, already-existing health resources. Following pilot social research on culturally acceptable approaches to the communities, interventions were designed through consultations with MOH officials and village leaders, and three interventions were implemented in cells 1–3, while cell 4 maintained standard MOH fixed-service-point approach for comparison.

Cell 1 tested the *zurugelu* ("togetherness") intervention, whereby traditional village structures are used to create health-care action committees with community-chosen health volunteers to aid in planning and delivering health services.

Cell 2 tested the MOH mobilization intervention, whereby service providers are relocated from fixed clinics to village residencies and assigned doorstep service delivery responsibilities.

Cell 3 tested a combination of the *zurugelu* and MOH interventions, allowing MOH professionalism to complement community accountability and sustainability.

Research results used to inform policy

Data was collected by the Navrongo Demographic Surveillance System to investigate the impact of the four service systems on child mortality and fertility practices. The most significant impact on child mortality was observed in the MOH mobilization cell, with a nearly 60% reduction of mortality for children exposed to the intervention for more than two years. This indicates the benefit of relocating trained nurses to village residences for improved access to and use of health services over time.

Changes in contraceptive use and fertility levels were most pronounced in the combined-intervention cell, where the project saw a reduction of the total fertility rate by one birth, a 15% decline, in comparison with control areas over three years. These results suggest that supply-side policies such as this combined community- and MOH-mobilization strategy can be effective in rural traditional communities.

As a direct result of the study results, the Ghanaian government incorporated Community Health and Planning Services (CHPS) into its latest five-year development plan. In a preliminary report of the health sector financing discussion group, policy-makers agreed on the benefits:

"Since experience from the field has shown that CHPS is the most cost-effective way of reducing the unnecessary morbidity and mortality responsible for Ghana's unacceptably high infant and maternal mortality rates, the group feels that allocating 6% of the proposed 2003 budget is reasonable and cost-effective," the Health Sector Financing Group concluded.

Source: www.navrongo.org

ation studies will be required in a number of different low-income countries. According to Haines et al. *(3)*:

- to better understand how interventions work or why they do not, qualitative approaches may need to be developed;
- refining interventions to be tested through preparatory research may increase the likelihood of effectiveness;
- assessing the operational costs of an intervention and its consequences in terms of savings or extra expenditures for providers and users of health-care services will require an economic evaluation.

The authors write: "The lack of rigorous evaluations of implementation strategies, particularly in low-income countries, reflects in part the low priority accorded to health services and systems research. Many stakeholders involved in implementing public health interventions do not appear to perceive investment in rigorous evaluation to be a priority. They believe they know what should be done, and their main priority is to put their beliefs into practice. In doing so the opportunity to generate robust evidence about how to change policy and practice is lost".

Also lost is the opportunity to gain valuable information about the people who are the targets of the intervention or programmes. This is true in both instances of successes and failures. When implementing research aimed at improving public health outcomes, it is crucial to understand the people who are meant to benefit from (or participate in) the research, be they policy-makers, health professionals or members of the public. Many research planners at national and global level often assume that there is nothing much to know about the target group, or that all that needs to be done is a short-term feasibility study. Evaluations into why projects have failed show this view is often wrong and can have important consequences for the outcomes of the project (see Box 4.12 for an illustrative example)

Community participation is essential

Programmes can be local, national or international in scale but what is critical to success in terms of improving health is how they function at the local level. Encouraging the use of existing knowledge to improve health depends on acquiring knowledge about how health and illness is regarded in any given community. Box 4.13 gives an example from Nepal of a rigorously designed study which found that community-based intervention involving women's groups significantly reduced neonatal mortality *(38)*.

Throughout this report, the case has been made for the fundamental importance of a strong local health system to the health and well-being of individuals, families, communities, nations and the world. But across the developing world, health-care systems are weak, and in some cases, barely functional. All major initiatives focusing on single diseases or conditions quickly run up against this harsh reality when they try to roll out their programmes. Since it would be

Box 4.12 Why research fails? A letter from an anthropologist

A widespread view among national and international public health care planners and managers is that most of what one needs to know is either known already or can be discerned through short-term feasibility studies. Health policies are designed along common international principles, but the question of why the health professionals and the public do not always respond is rarely tackled or taken seriously. This is a major knowledge gap. I will give an example to illustrate my point.

I was involved in a reproductive health and family planning project in Egypt where one of the tasks was to establish a referral system. Despite a huge effort on our part we failed. There were virtually no referrals from physicians in primary care. Physicians, specialists and health officials suggested more training was needed to solve the problem but they did not even consider that there might be an underlying problem.

I decided to conduct some research of my own which I termed 'Finding Underlying Causes for Failure of Referral System'. To cut a long story short, the cause was very simple: primary care physicians were afraid that referring patients meant they would lose their professional credibility as doctors.

For the patients, being referred meant that the doctor did not know and so he ran the risk of losing his patients. In a society where healing powers are connected with personal power, this behaviour is perfectly logical. Instead of being referred, the women went to the next doctor when the first doctor's prescriptions did not help, and so on.

When the problem was addressed in subsequent workshops, everyone admitted that this was indeed the root of problem and that behavioural change needed to be addressed to overcome this problem.

The notion of healing as a personal ability is common in many societies in the developing world and may have hampered many projects. But more often than not this issue may not have been taken into account in the design of a study. There are many other culture-specific notions that are vital for behavioural change with regard to health.

Research in this field is difficult, time-consuming and costly. However, if any aspect of a project fails, we need to scrutinize the underlying causes through research and not—as is common practice—to vaguely call for a "new approach". A pool of valuable results from all over the world could then contribute to the knowledge base and improve the chances of success in future.

Source: Letter from Dr Irene Leverenz, Berlin, Germany, April 2, 2004.

unethical to wait for a country to have a well-regulated, transparent and functioning health system before attempting to use knowledge to improve health, "creative" solutions must be found. Given that many people in low-income countries purchase medicines from local vendors and self-treat before considering a visit to a health-care provider sometimes working in an unregulated private practice, community-based approaches to programme implementation are common. There have been some remarkable success stories.

The introduction of oral rehydration therapy (ORT) in Bangladesh is a classic example *(39)*. In the late 1960s a group of public health doctors were sent on a mission to treat people living in a remote area of Bangladesh afflicted with dysentery. After many trips to the village with heavy backpacks containing intravenous rehydration solution, they sought new ways to address this common problem. Basic research had shown the importance of salt to avoid dehydration and the role of sugar in absorbing water and salt through the intestinal wall. Researchers at the International Center for Diarrhoeal Disease Research in Bangladesh developed variations and refinements of oral rehydration solutions and conducted trials on the efficacy of this relatively simple treatment. BRAC, one of the world's largest NGOs, discovered how to make the solution with common household items. In the 1980s, with government backing, BRAC launched a nationwide health campaign to teach mothers in rural areas how to prepare and administer ORT, a simple solution of water, sugar and salt, for use against diarrhoeal disease (see Figure 4.3). Social marketing and army-like

Box 4.13 Community participation in health research: an example from Nepal

Neonatal deaths in poor rural populations can be reduced significantly by simple, cost-effective measures involving women's groups in local communities, a recently published study conducted in Nepal has shown.

Neonatal deaths are a major public health concern in much of the developing world. Of the four million neonatal deaths which are reported every year, 98% occur in developing countries. In India, for example, 70% of infant mortality is due to babies dying in the neonatal period of their lives. In Nepal, 90% of deliveries in the poorest households occur at home. Logically, community participation would seem to be an effective approach to reduce neonatal mortality in this resource-poor setting.

Based on a randomized controlled trial design, the study involved 12 cluster pairs: one was the intervention arm and the other the control arm. Village development committees and women's groups in villages were closely involved in the study's design and implementation. A facilitator worked with the women's groups in monthly meetings using innovative participatory learning strategies. The researchers took an "action-learning" approach where local perinatal problems were identified and strategies collectively formulated, implemented and assessed.

During the trial, which was conducted from 2001 to 2003, there was a significant reduction in the neonatal mortality rate in 11 out of the 12 intervention clusters compared with that of the control groups (see figure). The rate in the intervention group was nearly 30% lower than in the control groups. In addition, the maternal mortality ratio was 69 per 100,000 in the intervention clusters compared to 341 per 100,000 in the control clusters. Women in the intervention group were also more likely to seek antenatal care and give birth in a hygienic institutional setting with the assistance of a trained birth attendant compared to the control group. The study illustrates the importance of community participation in health research. Moreover, this is an intervention which is potentially sustainable, scalable and transferable to other developing countries.

Neonatal mortality rates in intervention and control cluster pairs

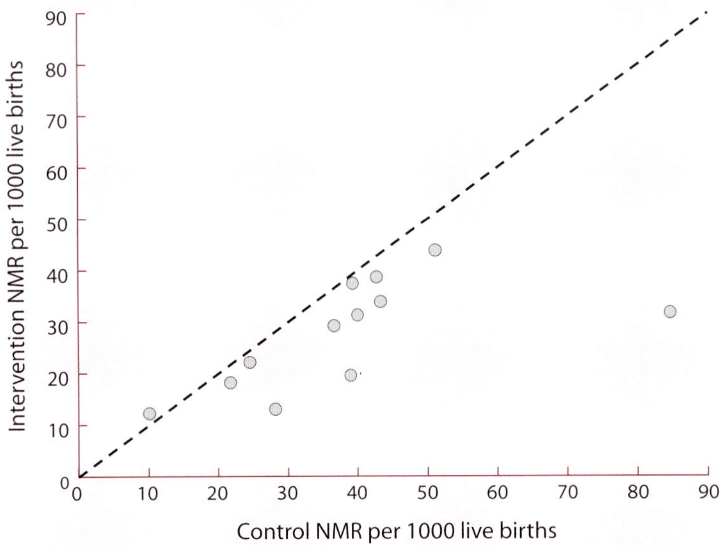

NMR=neonatal mortality rate. Dotted line is line of equality

Source: Manandhar DS et al. Effect of a participatory intervention with women's groups on birth outcomes in Nepal: cluster-randomised controlled trial. *Lancet*, 2004, 364:970–979.

logistics helped to ensure the success of the campaign. Having reached over 90% of all households, ORT has contributed to a significant decline in infant morbidity and mortality in Bangladesh. The *Lancet* has described ORT as "potentially the most important medical advance of this century", and UNICEF built on this success story and incorporated ORT as a key component to its "child survival and development revolution".

The African Programme for Onchocerciasis Control is another example highlighting the importance of community participation in disease control. A recent evaluation concluded that community-directed treatment is a feasible and effective means of ivermectin delivery for the treatment of onchocerciasis (see Box 4.14). The strategy, which is now being considered as a model in

Figure 4.3 Simple solutions: treating diarrhoea in Bangladesh

(a) A mother in a Bangladesh village preparing a lobon-gur (salt-local brown sugar) solution under the watchful eyes of a trained health worker.

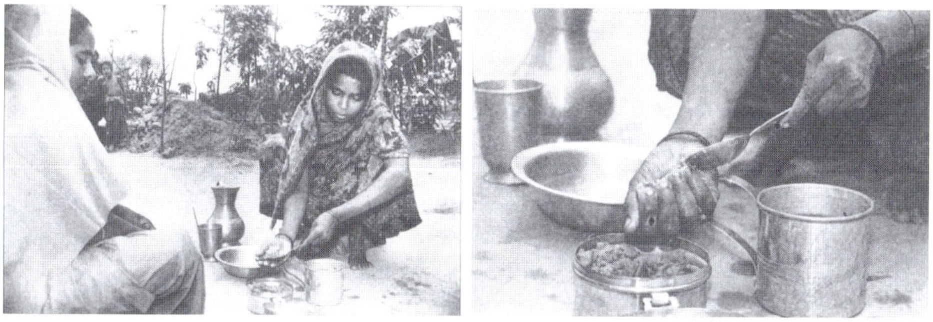

(b) A child with diarrhoea drinks the lobon-gur solution.

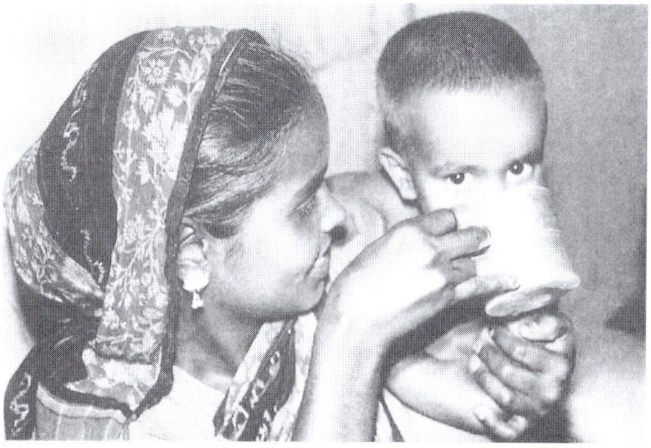

Source: Chowdhury AMR, Cash R. *A simple solution-teaching millions to treat diarrhoea at home.* Dhaka, University Press Limited, 1996.

developing other community-based programmes, is based of the following underlying principles *(40)*:

- Communities are powerful influencers of acceptance and change in much of the developing world, arguably much more so than in the developed world.
- Implementing a programme without the acceptance and explicit support of community leaders is probably doomed to fail.
- Health research should include households and community-based care in the private and informal sectors.

Regional perspective 7

Research on how to improve community and grassroots participation in health systems research should be given high priority.

Box 4.14 Research for control: the onchocerciasis experience

Two decades ago, onchocerciasis, or river blindness, was a major public health threat that devastated socioeconomic development in West Africa. Onchocerciasis is a parasitic disease transmitted to humans by blackflies who live near rivers. Although the disease is rarely fatal, it causes severe itching, skin lesions and in advanced cases, blindness. It is the world's second leading infectious cause of blindness. While approximately 18 million people are still estimated to be infected—more than 99% of whom live in Africa—tremendous success in controlling this debilitating disease has been made in recent years, thanks largely to two research-focused programmes, the Onchocerciasis Control Programme (OCP) and the African Programme for Onchocerciasis Control (APOC). The great strides made in treatment by these two programmes have been so significant that onchocerciasis is no longer classified as a significant public health problem.

Both OCP and APOC have capitalized on epidemiological research and rapid assessment methods in endemic areas to identify target areas for treatment as quickly as possible. For example, community trials of ivermectin, the primary drug used to treat onchocerciasis, helped to define cost-effective control strategies, just as Community-Directed Treatments have helped to ensure effective and sustainable ivermectin treatment. Modelling research was also employed to predict treatment needs for future onchocerciasis trends.

Perhaps the most useful application of onchocerciasis research has been the implementation of community diagnosis and self-directed treatment. By providing communities with the essential tools to both diagnose and treat onchocerciasis, the research community has not only greatly diminished the threat of onchocerciasis as a public health risk, but also made the communities at risk themselves self-sufficient.

Ongoing research continues to refine the process by which communities are able to treat themselves for onchocerciasis. For instance, the development of RAPLOA, a quick diagnostic test to determine a community's level of loa loa or eye-worm infection is ultimately a tool that will further accelerate onchocerciasis treatment. This is because people who are heavily infected with loa loa are at risk of neurological damage if treated with ivermectin, which is used to treat onchocerciasis. African researchers recently developed a questionnaire which health surveyors can use to rapidly determine whether communities are suitable for self-directed treatment. Thus, in communities where more than 40% of the population is found to have had a history of loa loa infection, onchocerciasis treatment can only be conducted under increased medical surveillance. RAPLOA was recently approved for use by APOC and has already been tested in four countries. It is this kind of practical research that has been most responsible for the rapid implementation of onchocerciasis treatment.

That the vast majority of onchocerciasis research has been conducted on the continent where it is most prevalent has also been a major factor in accelerating the operational benefits of such research initiatives. More than 95% of the researchers involved in onchocerciasis have been African scientists.

The onchocerciasis experience illustrates the importance of research that is driven primarily by clinical application. By focusing onchocerciasis studies on tools that might quickly be adopted by affected communities, scientists have recognized that public health threats will be addressed more quickly with public participation.

Community-directed Treatment (ComDT)

In ComDT it is the community itself rather than the health services that directs the treatment process. The community decides collectively:

- whether they want invermectin treatment;
- how invermectin tablets will be collected from the medical store;
- when it will be distributed;
- how it will be distributed;
- who in the community will be responsible for the distribution and record keeping;
- how the community will monitor the process.

The health workers only provide the necessary training and supervision.

Source: Remme JHF. Research for control: the onchocerciasis experience. *Tropical Medicine and International Health*, 2004, 9(2):243–254.

4.7 Summary

Very little is known about how best to facilitate the use of research in developing countries. One of the three main messages of *Knowledge for Better Health* is that it is not only a question of using what is already known, but also of doing more research to learn how to bridge this gap. The case studies presented in this chapter have illustrated how the combination of research and action can succeed in improving health systems, health outcomes and health equity.

Programmes and policies aimed at improving health need to be grounded in appropriate research conducted in the real world of competing priorities and realities. It is unrealistic to expect that every country can participate in the discovery of new treatments and diagnostics. But every country should engage in health systems research, which primarily seeks to improve the equitable delivery of health care for everyone.

References

1. Haines A, Donald A (eds). *Getting research findings into practice*. London, BMJ Books, 2nd edition, 2002.
2. Getting research to policy and practice. In: *Strengthening Health Systems: The role and promise of policy and systems research*, Geneva, Alliance for Health Policy and Systems Research, 2004.
3. Haines A et al. Bridging the implementation gap between knowledge and action for health. *Bulletin of the World Health Organization*, 2004, 82:724–732.
4. Jha P et al. Improving the health of the global poor. *Science*, 2002, 295:2036–2039.
5. Lenfant C. Clinical research to clinical practice: Lost in translation. *New England Journal of Medicine*, 2003, 349:868–874.
6. *Crossing the quality chasm: a new health system for the 21st century*. Washington, DC, Institute of Medicine, 2001.
7. Jones G et al. How many child deaths can we prevent this year. *Lancet*, 2003, 362:65–71
8. ASPAC Collaborative Group. Asia-Pacific Collaboration on Coronary Heart Disease Risk Factor Intervention: Study Design and Methods. *Heart, Lung and Circulation*, 2001, 10:24–29.
9. Attaran A. WHO, the Global Fund, and medical malpractice in malaria treatment. *Lancet*, 2004, 363:237–240.
10. Peckham M, Smith R. *Scientific basis of health services*. London, BMJ Publishing Group, 1996.
11. Moynihan R. Using health research in policy and practice: case studies in nine countries. New York, NY, Milbank Memorial Fund, 2004.
12. *What's worked? Accounting for success in global health*. Washington, DC, Center for Global Development, in press, 2005.
13. Lomas J. Retailing research: increasing the role of evidence in clinical services for childbirth. *The Milbank Quarterly*, 1993, 71:439–75.
14. Lavis et al, Examining the role of health services research in public policymaking. *The Milbank Quarterly*, 2002; 80:125–154.
15. Bensing JM et al. Doing the right thing and doing it right: toward a framework for assessing the policy relevance of health services research. *International Journal of Technology Assessment in Health Care*, 2003, 19:604–612.
16. Garner P et al. Implementing research findings in developing countries. *British Medical Journal*, 1998, 317:531–535.
17. Lavis J et al. How can research organizations more effectively transfer research knowledge to decision makers. *Milbank Quarterly*, 2003, 81:221–248.
18. Black RE, Morris SS, Bryce J. Where and why are 10 million children dying every year? *Lancet*, 2003, 361:2226–2234.
19. Bryce J et al. Multi-Country Evaluation of IMCI Study Group. *Lancet*, 2003, 362:159–164.
20. Victora CG et al. Applying an equity lens to child health and mortality: More of the same is not enough. *Lancet*, 2003, 362:233–241.
21. Bellagio Study Group on Child Survival. Knowledge into action for child survival. *Lancet*, 2003, 362:323–327.
22. Black N. Public accountability: One rule for practitioners, one for scientists? *Journal of Health Services Research and Policy*, 2001, 6:131–132.

23. Frenk J. Balancing relevance and excellence: organizational responses to link research with decision making. *Social Science and Medicine*, 1992, 35:1397–1404.
24. Berwick D. Disseminating innovations in health care. *Journal of the American Medical Association*, 2003, 289:1969–1975.
25. Berwick DM, Nolan TW. Physicians as leaders in improving health care: a new series in Annals of Internal Medicine. *Annals of Internal Medicine*, 1998, 128:289–92.
26. Davis D et al. The case for knowledge translation: shortening the journey from evidence to effect. *British Medical Journal*, 2003, 327:33–5.
27. Page J et al. Attitudes of developing world physicians to where medical research is performed and reported. *BMC Public Health*, 2003, 3:6.
28. Lomas J et al. On being a good listener: Setting priorities for applied health services research. *Milbank Quarterly*, 2003, 81:363–388.
29. Oxman AD et al. Users' guides: VI: How to use an overview. *Journal of the American Medical Association*, 1994, 272:1367–1371.
30. Grimshaw J et al. Systematic review of guideline dissemination and implementation strategies. Abstract O-22. XI Cochrane Colloquium, Barcelona, Spain, 27–31 October 2003.
31. Hanney SR et al. The utilisation of health research in policy-making: concepts, examples and methods of assessment. *Health Research Policy and Systems*, 2003, 1:2.
32. Innvaer S et al. Health policy-makers' perceptions of their use of evidence: A systematic review. *Journal of Health Services Research and Policy*, 2002, 7:239–244.
33. Canadian Health Services Research Foundation. 2001. Is Research Working for You? A Self Assessment Tool. Version 3. Ottawa, Canadian Health Services Research Foundation.
34. Andersen KS. The reforming states group and the promotion of federalism. *Milbank Quarterly*, 1998, 76:103–136.
35. Andreano R. *The international health policy programme—an internal assessment*. Madison, WI, University of Wisconsin Press for the International Health Policy Program, 2001.
36. Batt K et al. The costs, effects and cost-effectiveness of strategies to increase coverage of routine immunizations in low- and middle-income countries: systematic review of the grey literature. *Bulletin of the World Health Organization*, 2004, 82:689–696.
37. Bryce J et al. The multi-country evaluation of the integrated management of childhood illness strategy: lessons for the evaluation of public health interventions. *American Journal of Public Health*, 2004, 94:406–415.
38. Manandhar DS et al. Effect of a participatory intervention with women's groups on birth outcomes in Nepal: cluster-randomised controlled trial. *Lancet*, 2004, 364:970–979.
39. Chowdhury AMR, Cash RA. *A simple solution—teaching millions to treat diarrhoea at home*. Dhaka, University Press Limited, 1996.
40. Remme JHF. Research for control: the onchocerciasis experience. *Tropical Medicine and International Health*, 2004, 9:243–254.

5

Recommendations and Action Plan

"Now is the time to make it happen where it matters, by turning scientific knowledge into effective action for people's health."
(Jong-Wook Lee)

"Knowing is not enough, we must apply; willing is not enough, we must act."
(Johann Wolfgang von Goethe)

5.1 Recommendations

Knowledge for Better Health reaffirms the view that the generation and application of high-quality knowledge is vital to a high performance health system and the socioeconomic development of any given country.

In order for national health research systems to effectively utilize knowledge to improve their performance, they should:

- be based on the principles of ethical practice and transparency, and focused on achieving health equity;
- be able to obtain and sustain public trust, confidence and support;
- be able to access and communicate reliable and relevant evidence, knowledge and information;
- be adequately financed and supported by strong and sustainable human and institutional capacities;
- be closely tied to the national health system, and be able to set research priorities and influence the research agenda;
- be strongly focused on narrowing the gap between what we have the knowledge to do and what is actually done, and on developing a culture where decisions taken by policy-makers, health professionals and the public are based on evidence;
- be able to integrate learning, problem-solving and innovation within the system;

- be linked with and contribute to regional and international health and health research activities and agendas.

The report proposes the following recommendations:

1. More investment is needed in relatively under-funded areas of health research, especially for a new, innovative approach to research on health systems.
2. Management of health research should be strengthened if research is to contribute to strengthening health systems and to building public confidence and trust in science.
3. Stronger emphasis should be placed on translating knowledge into actions to improve health thereby bridging the gap between what is known and what is actually being done.

These recommendations take into account support for existing initiatives and past recommendations, as well as identifying future opportunities and new initiatives relevant to current challenges.

The recommendations of *Knowledge for Better Health* are at the heart of the report's action plan, which is outlined in the following section. It is now a matter of urgency to make health systems the focus of national and international efforts in order to improve their ability to provide health care in an equitable fashion.

5.2 ACTION PLAN

The key components of the action plan are summarized in Table 5.1 and described in more detail below. The eleven-point action plan includes examples of both ongoing and planned initiatives in the three recommendation areas. By no means an exhaustive list, its aim is to highlight activities at the national, regional and global level that address the recommendations in an effective and targeted manner.

INCREASE INVESTMENTS IN HEALTH RESEARCH

1. **The "grand challenge" of health systems research:** A major programme along the lines of a "grand challenge in global public health" (see reference 24 in Chapter 2) is urgently needed to support research which may improve delivery and achievement of high and equitable coverage of health services. The level of support for such a programme must be substantially higher than what has been spent on this field of research to date. Countries and international agencies must focus on important areas such as research into equity issues including gender, community participation in health research and operational studies on health systems. At the same time, the programme should also promote and encourage the more "fundamental" and "frontier" areas of health systems research.

Table 5.1 Action plan overview

Recommendation	*Action items and initiatives**
Increase investments in health research	■ Programme to support health systems research (1) ■ Financing health research (2) ■ New diagnostics, vaccines and therapeutics (3)
Strengthen management of health research systems	■ Access to information (4) ■ International clinical trials register (5) ■ Ethical health research (6) ■ Benchmark national health research systems towards health goals (7) ■ Regional and global alliances for research governance (8)
Bridge the gap between knowledge and action	■ Evidence-informed policy and practice (9) ■ Use of evidence by national policy-makers in decision-making (10) ■ Basic health information (11)

* Numbers in brackets refer to the 11 action items and initiatives listed in Section 5.2.

Source: World Health Organization, 2004.

It should also include research into outcomes of health system reforms and development of standardized indicators to monitor performance. Focus must be placed on strengthening health systems so that they are able to deal with the dual threat of both communicable and noncommunicable diseases. Initiatives such as the Alliance for Health Policy and Systems Research and linked networks of institutions serving as regional research and training centres on health systems research should be evaluated and strengthened.

2. **Financing health research:** As first proposed by the Commission on Health Research and Development in 1990, countries should allocate at least 2% of national health expenditure and 5% of health project assistance to health research. This should include an effort to monitor health research spending within national health accounts (NHA). Countries also need to explore more innovative ways to finance health research. Some countries have introduced a "sin" tax which allocates a proportion of tax revenue from gambling, alcohol and tobacco sales to health promotion and research. On a global level, major supporters of health research must renew their commitment to reduce the 10/90 gap.

3. **New diagnostics, vaccines and therapeutics:** There is a need to continue to promote the role of public-private partnerships and other innovative approaches in addressing the neglected diseases that mainly affect the poor. The development of priority diagnostics, vaccines and therapeutics should be a priority. Consideration should also be given to analysing issues such as tax relief schemes and other financial incentives within the existing patent system. Other novel approaches such as the "open source" approach to research should also be evaluated.

Strengthen management of health research systems

4. **Information access:** (i) There are a number of initiatives that promote access to reliable health information and research (both primary and secondary) such as BIREME (Latin American and Caribbean Center on Health Sciences Information), the Cochrane Collaboration, HEN (Health Evidence Network), HINARI (Health InterNetwork Access to Research Initiative), INCLEN's (International Clinical Epidemiology Network) Knowledge Plus Project, the Ptolemy project to improve access to health information in Africa, and SHARED (Scientists for Health and Research for Development) as well as "open access" journals. These should all be promoted, expanded and allocated more funding. Where appropriate, such initiatives should also consider non-Internet based strategies, such as CD-ROMS, and advances in information technology such as Wi-Fi connectivity; (ii) developing countries should also invest in increasing the number of national and regional health and medical journals, as well as in improving their quality and expanding distribution. It is necessary to improve editorial and managerial skills, support peer review processes and boost access to these publications (e.g. through a web presence, full text electronic versions and CD-ROMS); (iii) the use of electronic information and communication technologies in health can help health professionals not only to keep pace with the latest scientific findings but also provide health professionals and lay persons with high-quality and relevant data. This can facilitate learning by removing distance and time barriers to the flow of information and knowledge for health. WHO's E-Health initiative could play a major role in providing people in developing countries with reliable web-based health information by facilitating the use of information to improve health; (iv) a global initiative should be launched to improve access to health-care and health research information in the developing world, led by WHO and its partners. The initiative could consider drafting a declaration of universal access to relevant, reliable and up-to-date health-care and health research information.

5. **International clinical trials register:** Responding to intense current interest in this issue, wide-ranging consultations on the establishment of an international clinical trials register are urgently needed. These consultations should include all interested stakeholders including research organizations, journal editors, consumer groups, funders and industry. A register could make information on clinical trials more easily accessible and would facilitate the recruitment of patients, and also help reduce duplication and publication bias. By improving the efficiency and transparency of the research process, such a register would address major contemporary ethical concerns and also help to build public confidence in science. Information contained in such a register would facilitate international collaboration in specific areas, capacity building activities in countries and public education about clinical research. In the longer term, a strengthened evidence base on such

trials will help in the formulation of policy pertaining to health services interventions. National registers of trials taking place in countries should also be established, perhaps led by national ethical review boards.

6. **Ethical research:** Countries should invest in building national capacity for the ethical review of health research. This fast evolving area has an impact on issues like human rights, justice, fairness, confidentiality, discrimination and stigmatization. At the global level, international organizations and donor agencies should consider allocating resources to help build such capacity in countries. The role of regional forums for improving ethical review capacity, such as FERCAP (Forum for Ethical Review Committees in Asian and Western Pacific region) and PABIN (Pan-African Bioethics Initiative), should be considered. At the same time, many researchers and research institutions in the developing world feel disadvantaged when entering into research collaborations with partners in the developed world. They have little say in determining priorities, are often treated as mere "specimen collectors" and do not share in the financial and intellectual benefits of the research. In clinical research, participants often have limited education or are illiterate and are sometimes coerced into participating in clinical trials. They are often not fully informed of their rights and of the risks involved, and sometimes not told of the results, or given the chance to benefit from the findings of the trial. In recognition of such potential problems, international agencies should consider establishing an international code of conduct for equitable partnerships in health research.

7. **Benchmark national health research systems towards health goals:** As an important managerial tool, countries should give priority to the development of indicators and a national process with many stakeholders, to describe, analyse and monitor health research systems to make these move toward health goals. The aim would be to provide indicators on all key functions and processes within health research systems, such as leadership, ethics, financing, human and institutional collaboration, information sharing, synthesis, and access on a range of research outputs not limited to scientific publications. WHO's Health Research Systems Analyses initiative is developing and testing this approach involving national task forces in 13 low- and middle-income countries. These task forces discuss how to institutionalize on-going monitoring, and its relevance to national policy-making and to health systems needs. Experiences gained are also shared across countries and at the regional level. Focusing more specifically on one key dimension of health research systems, there is also a dearth of reliable information on the number of people working in health research in many low- and middle-income countries. Arguably, some of these countries do not have enough skilled staff to maintain even a minimal health research system. More reliable data and analysis are needed to help develop incentives for health researchers in developing countries to make staying at home

attractive and lucrative. International agencies and initiatives involved in workforce migration issues need to do more to address these challenges.

8. **Regional and global alliances for research governance:** Regional health research forums in Asia, Africa, Latin America and other regions were established following the International Conference on Health Research for Development in Bangkok in 2000. Their role should be more clearly defined and their activities given more support. The conference also proposed setting up a global coalition for health research. These entities and other forms of alliances or coalitions involving national health research councils, major research institutions or agencies from developed and developing countries need to be critically assessed to ensure their unique and value-added contributions. More recently, the Research Agency Collaborative for Global Health (REACH) proposed the creation of a network of national research agencies with the broad aim of increasing research on the health problems of low- and middle-income countries and simultaneously contribute to research capacity building in these countries. An idea for a Forum of Health Research and Development Partners has also been mooted. This would be a forum for research agencies, development agencies, donors and industry players to improve coordination of their activities and prevent duplication of the research they support in developing countries. Such a forum could consider models of collaboration and coordination, as well as potential initiatives in various areas of health research.

Bridging the gap between knowledge and action

9. **Evidence-informed policy and practice:** Several ongoing initiatives in this area should be promoted and provided with more support. These include: the Agency for Healthcare Research and Quality's Evidence-based Practice Centres Programme (EPC), the Alliance for Health Policy and Systems Research (AHPSR), Cochrane Collaboration's Effective Practice and Organization of Care Group (EPOC), European Observatory for Health Systems and Policies, GRADE (Grading of Recommendations Assessment, Development and Evaluation) Working Group, HEN, International Network of Agencies on Health Technology Assessment (INAHTA), INCLEN's Knowledge Plus Project, and the United Kingdom's National Institute for Clinical Excellence (NICE). Countries should also develop the skills to synthesize research and evidence to help them reach the conclusions that can help to shape policy, improve healthcare and better educate the public. Such skills should be acknowledged as crucial and as a legitimate form of research, and appropriately rewarded. Systematic reviews of existing research should inform decisions on whether to finance further research. A similar approach should also be taken in the development of policy, technical and practice recommendations, including those put forward by WHO. At the global level, more should be invested in improving the quality and

coverage of existing databases of research information including those in languages other than English. The publication of systematic reviews as bona fide scientific articles should also be encouraged. Additionally, more systematic reviews of health problems in developing countries should be carried out, and methodologies for performing such reviews beyond clinical trials should be improved. Short research and policy briefs for policy-makers based on research syntheses and systematic reviews should be promoted.

10. **Use of evidence by national policy-makers in decision-making**: The use of sound evidence to develop health policies at all levels should be practised by all countries. Systems should be created whereby evidence-based advice is relayed to government policy-makers. This could include the training of intermediaries who could communicate researchers' data to policy-makers. Other players, such as parliamentarians, the media and civil society, could also be involved in the process of translating research data into policy. The need is especially acute in developing countries due to sometimes limited access to information and scarce capacity for knowledge translation. An initiative that builds on previous efforts should be launched with support from governments, donors and international organizations to try out various mechanisms that would effectively place evidence in the hands of policy-makers when making decisions in the health sector. Successful initiatives in the developed world, such as the Reforming States Group and the European Observatory on Health Systems and Policies, could potentially serve as models for national decision-making in low- and middle-income countries. An analogous "Reforming Nations Group" should be established in regions of greatest need.

11. **Basic health information**: Countries need to make a concerted effort to build capacity for generating and disseminating reliable and accurate basic health information at the district and national level, and to integrate data collection and analysis within national health systems. This is vital in order to overcome the lack of access to such information on health in many developing countries. This basic health information should cover areas such as mortality, morbidity, disease incidence and prevalence, equity and coverage of health-care interventions and quality of service delivery. It should also include data relevant to scaling up treatment and prevention programmes. Moreover, there is a critical need for data that describe the performance of health systems and critical dimensions of health systems functions (e.g. financing, human resources and service delivery), in addition to information on health research systems mentioned above. The newly formed Health Metrics Network at WHO is an effective international vehicle for providing more accurate and reliable health information. Successful models like INDEPTH (International Network for the Continuous Demographic Evaluation of Populations and Their Health in Developing Countries) need to be supported and promoted.

Glossary of Terms

Applied research	Original investigation undertaken in order to acquire new knowledge but directed primarily towards a specific practical aim or objective.
Basic research	Experimental or theoretical work undertaken primarily to acquire new knowledge of the underlying foundation of phenomena and observable facts, with no particular application or use in view.
Benchmarking	A process of measuring another organization's product or service according to specified standards in order to compare it with and improve one's own product or service.
Burden of disease	Days lost through sickness and disability and years of life lost through the same.
Equality	Principle by which all persons or things under consideration are treated in the same way.
Equity	Principle of being fair to all persons, with reference to a defined and recognized set of values.
Grey literature	A range of published and unpublished material that is not normally identifiable through conventional methods of bibliographic control.
Health research system	The people, institutions, and activities that act together to generate high-quality knowledge that can be used to promote, restore, and/or maintain the health status of populations. It should include mechanisms to encourage the use of research.
Health system	The people, institutions, and resources that operate as a whole to provide health care and improve the health of the population it serves.

Health systems research	The production of new knowledge and applications to improve the way societies organize themselves to achieve health goals. It includes how societies plan, manage, and finance activities to improve health and takes into consideration the roles, perspectives, and interests of different actors. The health system's functions of regulation, organization, financing, and delivery of services are the focal subjects. It is often understood to include health policy research.
Inequality in health	Differences in health status across individuals in the population.
Inequity in health	The systematic and potentially remediable differences in one or more aspects of health across socially, economically, demographically, or geographically defined population groups or subgroups.
Knowledge management	A set of principles and tools to optimize and integrate the processes of creating, sharing and using knowledge. The overall aim is to solve problems and improve organizational effectiveness in the field of public health.
Knowledge translation	The exchange, synthesis, and effective communication of reliable and relevant research results. The focus is on promoting interaction among the producers and users of research, removing the barriers to research use, and tailoring information to different target audiences so that effective interventions are used more widely.
National health accounts	Information, usually in the form of indicators, a country may collect on its health expenditures. Indicators may include total health expenditure, public expenditure, private expenditure, out-of-pocket expenditure, tax-funded and other public expenditure, social security expenditure, and public expenditure on health.

Open access publication	When a peer reviewed research article is made universally and freely accessible via the Internet and deposited immediately upon publication, without embargo, in at least one widely and internationally recognized open access repository. Any third party has the right to reproduce the research article in its entirety or in part provided there is proper attribution of authorship and no substantive errors are introduced in the process.
Out-of-pocket payment	Fee paid by the consumer of health services directly to the provider.
Public health	The science and art of promoting health, preventing disease, and prolonging life through the organized efforts of society.
Research synthesis	The process through which two or more research studies are assessed with the objective of summarizing the evidence relating to a particular question. It is based on the principle that science is cumulative.
Strategic research	Research that has been identified at the time of funding to be of evident interest to a wide range of users.
System	A group of elements operating together to achieve a common goal.
Systematic reviews	A rigorous method of identifying, appraising, and synthesizing original research using strategies that limit bias and random error.
Translational research	The process of applying ideas, insights, and discoveries generated through basic scientific inquiry to the treatment or prevention of human disease.

Information Sources

The sources for data and information in the report are given on the *World Report on Knowledge for Better Health* website at www.who.int/rpc/wr2004. This includes information sources for quotations, the "Interesting numbers" featured at the beginning of each chapter, terms listed in the glossary and a full list of contributors to the report.

Sources for tables, figures, and boxes are given under each item.

Background documents

The web site also contains links to additional background documents that provided additional inputs to the Report. The following documents are available:

1. Report from a Partners Forum meeting in London, United Kingdom (April 27–28, 2004).
2. Reports and publications from the Task Force on Health Systems Research Priorities and the Task Force on Knowledge Access and Sharing.
3. Reports from regional consultations convened to obtain inputs for the report (March–May, 2004).
4. Report from a meeting on macroeconomic stability and scaling-up of aid to combat HIV/AIDS in low-income countries (London, June 22, 2004).
5. Report from a consultation with NGOs on health system research priorities (Durban, South Africa, June 12, 2004).
6. Report from a consultation with senior government policy-makers on the use of evidence in policy-making (Kuala Lumpur, Malaysia, September 16–17, 2004).
7. Report from a workshop on research priorities in human resources for health (Cape Town, South Africa, September 6–8, 2004).
8. Evidence gaps matrices prepared by WHO departments involved in key MDG areas (maternal health, child health, HIV/AIDS, tuberculosis, malaria).
9. A report entitled *Knowledge Gaps and Research Priorities Related to Health as Reflected in the Millennium Project's Task Force Documents* (by Margarita Hurtado).

10. History of health systems research in WHO (by Yvo Nuyens).
11. Selected key publications in various academic journals.
12. Essential reading list for Chapter 3 of the report on health research systems.
13. Other relevant documents.

RELATED PUBLICATIONS

In addition, several related publications will also become available at the time of the official release of the report:

1. *WHO Bulletin Special Issue* on the theme of Bridging the Know-do Gap in Global Health (October, 2004).
2. Collected series of articles in the *Lancet* on health research and health systems research.
3. *British Medical Journal* special issue on Learning from Developing Countries.
4. *Strengthening Health Systems: The role and promise of policy and systems research*, Geneva, Alliance for Health Policy and Systems Research, 2004. This is a biennial review of health systems research.
5. *The Global Forum Update on Research for Health 2005*. Geneva, Global Forum for Health Research, 2004. This publication consists of a collection of short articles from a wide range of people around the world, providing their views on the whole field of health research for development and closing the 10/90 gap.
6. Van Damme W et al. Health systems research and INCO-DEV: Lessons for the future. Preliminary report of Expert Team meeting, Brussels, February 9–13, 2004. (Full report to be published by the end of 2004).

Abbreviations and Acronyms

AHPSR	Alliance for Health Policy and Systems Research
ART	Antiretroviral therapy
BIREME	Latin American and Caribbean Center on Health Sciences Information
BRAC	Formerly known as Bangladesh Rural Advancement Committee
BSE	Bovine spongiform encephalopathy
CIAR	Canadian Institute of Advanced Research
CIHR	Canadian Institutes of Health Research
DALY	Disability adjusted life years
DNA	Deoxyribonucleic acid
DOTS	Directly Observed Treatment, Short Course strategy
ENHR	Essential National Health Research
GAVI	Global Alliance for Vaccines and Immunization
GCP	Good Clinical Practice
GDP	Gross domestic product
HEN	Health Evidence Network
HINARI	Health InterNetwork Access to Research Initiative
HMN	Health Metrics Network
HRH	Human resources for health
HRP	UNDP/UNFPA/WHO/World Bank Special Programme of Research, Development and Research Training in Human Reproduction
HRSA	Health Research System Analyses (initiative)
IMCI	Integrated Management of Childhood Illness
INAHTA	International Network of Agencies on Health Technology Assessment
INCLEN	International Clinical Epidemiology Network

INDEPTH	International Network for the Continuous Demographic Evaluation of Populations and Their Health in Developing Countries
ISI	Institute for Scientific Information
ISC	International Scientific Cooperation programme
ISRCTN	International Standard Randomized Controlled Trial Number
MDGs	Millennium Development Goals
NCD	Noncommunicable disease
NGO	Nongovernmental organization
NHA	National health accounts
NICE	National Institute for Clinical Excellence
OECD	Organisation for Economic Development and Cooperation
ORT	Oral rehydration therapy
PLoS	Public Library of Science
PLWA	People living with AIDS
PMTCT	Prevention of mother-to-child transmission of HIV/AIDS
PPP	Public-private partnerships
R&D	Research and development
REACH	Research Agency Collaborative for Global Health
RHL	Reproductive Health Library
RICYT	Ibero-American and Inter-American Network on Science and Technology Indicators
S&T	Science and technology
SARS	Severe Acute Respiratory Syndrome
SciELO	Scientific Electronic Library Online
TDR	UNICEF/UNDP/World Bank/WHO Special Programme for Research and Training in Tropical Diseases
TEHIP	Tanzania Essential Health Interventions Project
UNDP	United Nations Development Programme
UNFPA	United Nations Population Fund
UNICEF	United Nations Children's Fund
WHO	World Health Organization